GAMUTS
IN
ULTRASOUND

GAMUTS
IN
ULTRASOUND

MICHAEL R. WILLIAMSON, M.D.

Chief, Diagnostic Ultrasound
University of New Mexico
School of Medicine
Albuquerque, New Mexico

SUSAN L. WILLIAMSON, M.D.

Associate Professor of Radiology
University of New Mexico
School of Medicine
Albuquerque, New Mexico

W.B. SAUNDERS COMPANY
Harcourt Brace Jovanovich, Inc.

Philadelphia / London / Toronto / Montreal / Sydney / Tokyo

W. B. SAUNDERS COMPANY
Harcourt Brace Jovanovich, Inc.

The Curtis Center
Independence Square West
Philadelphia, Pennsylvania 19106-3399

Library of Congress Cataloging-in-Publication Data

Williamson, Michael R.
    Gamuts in ultrasound / Michael R. Williamson, Susan L. Williamson.
      p. cm.
    ISBN 0-7216-3544-X
    1. Diagnosis, Ultrasonic.   I. Williamson, Susan L.
  II. Title.
    [DNLM: 1. Ultrasonography—methods.   WB 289 W731g]
  RC78.7.U4W55   1992
  616.07′543—dc20
  DNLM/DLC
  for Library of Congress   91-35155
                                     CIP

Editor: Lisette Bralow
Designer: Joan Sinclair

GAMUTS IN ULTRASOUND   ISBN   0-7216-3544-X

Printed in Mexico

Last digit is the print number: 9   8   7   6   5   4   3   2   1

Preface

This book is patterned after similar works in general radiology and nuclear medicine. It is our hope that these gamuts will be useful to both physicians and ultrasonographers when that unusual or rare ultrasound finding occurs. Many of the gamuts are divided into "common" and "uncommon." However, in some instances the entities in a gamut may all be rare or may all be common. In those cases, we have not attempted to separate the items in the list into artificially created categories.

For several of the entries we have provided additional information in the form of brief comments. We have not attempted to do this for all entries, as that would greatly expand the size of the book. We only added comments when they might be helpful in distinguishing between similar entities or as a means of reducing the number of possible diagnoses. In addition, we have made an earnest attempt to use the sonographic terminology consistently when describing the appearance of these often obscure and confusing entities.

MICHAEL WILLIAMSON

Contents

UTERUS 56

OVARIES AND ADNEXA 59

ADRENAL GLANDS 65

KIDNEY 67

PART II   **OBSTETRICS**

PART III PEDIATRIC

PART I
ADULT

NECK

Masses

THYROID

Enlarged
Multiple nodules
Solitary nodules
Calcifications
Hypoechoic areas

BREAST

Cystic lesions
Masses
Shadowing from breast lesion

ABDOMINAL WALL

Masses

INTRAPERITONEAL, GENERAL

Masses
Fluid
Right lower quadrant cystic
   structure

AORTA

Displacement
Dilation
Periaortic fluid
Mass within

INFERIOR VENA CAVA

Echoes within
Displacement

LIVER

Hepatomegaly
Overall increased echogenicity
Decreased echogenicity
Bright periportal echoes (starry-sky
   liver)
Increased diameter of liver vessels
Intrahepatic shadowing
Cystic lesions, intrahepatic
Solid lesions, intrahepatic
Calcification in a focal hepatic
   lesion
Intrahepatic calcifications (no
   accompanying lesion)
Invasion of hepatic vessels by a
   mass
Lesion with echogenic rim

1

GALLBLADDER

Septae
Courvoisier gallbladder
    (overdistended)
Echoes within
Shadows from wall
Nonvisualization
Wall thickening
Pericholecystic fluid
Cysts within the wall

BILIARY SYSTEM

"Too many tubes" in the liver
Enlarged common duct
Echoes within the common duct
Echogenic bile duct wall

PANCREAS

Focal mass
Cystic lesions
Diffusely increased size
Echogenic
Hypoechoic
Decreased size
Peripancreatic hypoechoic masses
Calcifications

SPLEEN

Enlarged
Focal abnormalities
Cysts
Masses
Calcifications

STOMACH

Wall thickening
Masses

BOWEL

Wall thickening
Masses

PELVIS

Masses, male

BLADDER

Masses
Wall thickening

UTERUS

Enlarged
Masses
Thickened endometrium
Endometrial fluid
Endometrial shadowing

OVARIES AND ADNEXA

Enlarged
Cystic or complex ovary or
    adnexal mass
Pelvic masses during pregnancy
Adnexal calcifications
Solid adnexal mass

ADRENAL GLANDS

Masses
Cysts
Calcifications

KIDNEY

Enlarged bilaterally, smooth
    contour
Enlarged unilaterally, smooth
    contour
Enlarged unilaterally, multifocal
    lesions
Enlarged bilaterally, multifocal
    lesions
Small, unilateral, smooth contour
Small, bilateral, smooth contour
Cystic masses
Complex masses
Solid masses

Renal pelvic masses
Abnormal echogenicity
  Increased cortical echogenicity
    compared to medulla
  Increased echogenicity, no distinction between cortex and medulla
Echogenic medulla
Decreased cortical echogenicity
Internal echogenic areas
Dilated collecting system
Confused with dilated collecting system
Wall thickening of collecting system
Echoes within the collecting system
Enlarged renal vessels
Perirenal fluid

KIDNEY TRANSPLANT

Enlarged
Increased echogenicity
Perinephric fluid
Masses

RETROPERITONEUM

Masses
Cystic lesions

SCROTUM

Fluid and masses, extratesticular
Cystic mass, extratesticular

TESTES

Abnormal echogenicity
Enlarged testicle
Cysts
Enlarged epididymis
Calcification
Hypoechoic bands

PROSTATE

Cysts
Hypoechoic lesions
Calcifications
Echogenic lesion
Seminal vesicle abnormalities

Neck

MASSES

Common

	Comment
Nodal metastases	
Inflammatory adenopathy	Usually hypoechoic

Uncommon

Brachial cleft cysts	
Neck abscesses	Usually complex echogenicity
Parathyroid adenoma	Usually hypoechoic
Lateral pharyngoesophageal diverticulum	May see air within mass or fluid

---

Hayashi N, Tamaki N, Konishi J, et al.: Lateral pharyngoesophageal diverticulum simulating thyroid adenoma on sonography. J Clin Ultrasound 12:592, 1984.

Thyroid

ENLARGED

Common	Comment
Graves' disease	
Subacute thyroiditis (de Quervain's)	Areas of increased and decreased echogenicity
Chronic thyroiditis (Hashimoto's)	Areas of increased and decreased echogenicity

Uncommon

Acute thyroiditis	
Lymphadenoid goiter	
Riedel's struma	Also known as Riedel's thyroiditis
Lymphoma	Frequently unilateral
Anaplastic carcinoma	

Clair MR, Mandelblatt S, Baim RS, et al.: Sonographic features of acute suppurative thyroiditis. J Clin Ultrasound 11:222, 1983.

Hayashi N, Tamaki N, Konishi J, et al.: Sonography of Hashimoto's thyroiditis. J Clin Ultrasound 14:123, 1986.

Parulekar SG, Katzman RA: Primary malignant lymphoma of the thyroid: Sonographic appearance. J Clin Ultrasound 14:60, 1986.

MULTIPLE NODULES (HYPOECHOIC OR HYPERECHOIC)

Common	Comment
Multinodular goiter	
Subacute thyroiditis	
Chronic thyroiditis	
Multiple adenomas	May be same as multinodular goiter

Uncommon

Lymphoma
Anaplastic carcinoma

Parulekar SG, Katzman RA: Primary malignant lymphoma of the thyroid: Sonographic appearance. J Clin Ultrasound 14:60, 1986.

SOLITARY NODULES (HYPOECHOIC OR HYPERECHOIC)

Common	Comment
Adenoma	

Uncommon	
Papillary thyroid cancer	Usually solid, hypoechoic; occasionally cystic
Follicular thyroid cancer	
Metastases	
Parathyroid adenoma	May be intrathyroidal

CALCIFICATIONS

Common	Comment
Papillary carcinoma	Psammomatous calcifications
Follicular carcinoma	
Adenoma	

Uncommon	
Undifferentiated carcinoma	
Multinodular goiter	
Postinflammatory necrosis	
Posthemorrhagic necrosis	
Thyroid cysts	May have eggshell calcifications

HYPOECHOIC AREAS

Common	Comment
Subacute thyroiditis	Also known as de Quervain's thyroiditis
Hashimoto's thyroiditis	
Multinodular goiter	

Uncommon	
Acute thyroiditis	

Clair MR, Mandelblatt S, Baim RS, et al.: Sonographic features of acute suppurative thyroiditis. J Clin Ultrasound 11:222, 1983.

Tokuda Y, Kasagi K, Yasuhiro I, et al.: Sonography of subacute thyroiditis: Changes in the findings during the course of the disease. J Clin Ultrasound 18:21, 1990.

Breast

CYSTIC LESIONS

Common

Benign simple cysts
Breast carcinoma
Abscesses

Comment

From dilatation of ducts

Uncommon

Galactocele
Hematoma
Metastases

From recently lactating breast

Jackson VP: Role of US in breast imaging. Radiology 177:305, 1990.

MASSES

Common

Fibroadenoma

Ductal carcinoma

Comment

Frequently hypoechoic; may show
   enhanced through transmission
Frequent irregular border; two thirds
   have posterior shadowing; usually
   do not see microcalcifications

Uncommon

Cystosarcoma phyllodes
Hematoma
Abscess
Metastases
Lobular carcinoma of breast
Giant fibroadenoma
Hamartoma
Cysts

Usually adolescent females

Adler DD, Jeffries DO, Helvie MA: Sonographic features of breast hamartomas. J Ultrasound Med
   9:85, 1990.
Steinbock RT, Stomper PC, Meyer JE, et al.: The ultrasound appearance of giant fibroadenoma. J Clin
   Ultrasound 11:451, 1983.

SHADOWING FROM BREAST LESION

Fat necrosis
Foreign body
Lipoma
Galactocele
Fibrocystic disease
Granular cell tumor (myoblastoma)
Hamartoma

Adler DD, Jeffries DO, Helvie MA: Sonographic features of breast hamartomas. J Ultrasound Med 9:85, 1990.

Harper AP, Kelly-Fry E, Noe JS, et al.: Ultrasound in the evaluation of solid breast masses. Radiology 146:731, 1983.

Heywang SH, Lipsit ER, Glassman LM, et al.: Specificity of ultrasonography in the diagnosis of benign breast masses. J Ultrasound Med 3:453, 1984.

Scatarige JC, Hsiu JG, de la Torre R, et al.: Acoustic shadowing in benign granular cell tumor (myoblastoma) of the breast. J Ultrasound Med 6:545, 1987.

Abdominal Wall

MASSES

Common

	Comment
Abscesses	Complex
Hematoma	
Ventral hernia containing bowel	

Uncommon

Seroma	Cystic
Cellulitis	
Tumors	
Desmoid	
Malignant fibrous histiocytoma	
Urachal cyst	Between bladder apex and umbilicus
Endometrioma in cesarean section scar	

Bouvier JF, Pascaud E, Mailhes F, et al.: Urachal cyst in the adult: Ultrasound diagnosis. J Clin Ultrasound 12:48, 1984.

Vincent LM, Mittelstaedt CA: Sonographic demonstration of endometrioma arising in Cesarean scar. J Ultrasound Med 4:437, 1985.

Yeh HC, Rabinowitz JG, Rosenblum J: Complimentary role of CT and ultrasonography in the diagnosis of desmoid tumor of abdominal wall. Comput Radiol 6:275, 1982.

Intraperitoneal, General

MASSES

Common

Common	Comment
Hematoma	
Abscess	
Fluid in bowel	
Pseudocyst of pancreas	
Abnormal bowel	
Infarcted	Usually appears complex
Infected	
Infiltrated (lymphoma)	
Obstructed	
Hematoma in wall	
Barium within	Solid
Intussusception	Solid or complex
Lymphoma	
Fecaloma	Impacted patients
Malignancy	
Ovary	
Colon	
Pancreas	
Gastric	
Metastases	

Uncommon

Uncommon	Comment
Duplication cyst	
Mesenteric cyst	May be serous or chylous
Lymphocele	
Disseminated hydatid disease	
Complex ascites	
Abdominal tuberculosis	
Omental tuberculosis	
Crohn's disease	
Echinococcus	Usually cystic
Omental cyst	
Mesothelioma of omentum	
Left ventricular aneurysm	
Surgical transposition of ovary	To move ovary out of radiation field
Peritoneal inclusion cyst	

MASSES (Continued)

Uncommon (Continued)	*Comment*
Fat necrosis	May simulate mass
Leiomyomatosis peritoneales disseminata	Females only; multiple mesothelial nodules
Ovarian vein thrombophlebitis	Usually puerperal
Mucocele of appendix	Complex mass with calcified rim
Tuberculous peritonitis	
Cystic lymphangioma	
Cystic mesothelioma	

Akhan O, Demirkazik FB, Demirkazik A, et al.: Tuberculous peritonitis: Ultrasonic diagnosis. J Clin Ultrasound 18:711, 1990.

Athey PA, Hacken JB, Estrada R: Sonographic appearance of mucocele of the appendix. J Clin Ultrasound 12:333, 1984.

Brauner M, Buffard MD, Jeantils V, et al.: Sonography and computed tomography of macroscopic tuberculosis of the liver. J Clin Ultrasound 17:563, 1989.

Cancelmo RP: Sonographic demonstration of multilocular peritoneal inclusion cyst. J Clin Ultrasound 11:334, 1983.

Davies RP, Kennedy G, Chatterton BE: Noncystic appearance of intraperitoneal echinococcus on ultrasonic examination. J Clin Ultrasound 14:55, 1986.

Derchi LE, Musante F, Biggi E, et al.: Sonographic appearance of fecal masses. J Ultrasound Med 4:573, 1985.

Giyanani VL, Jackson MK, Gerlock AJ, et al.: Omental cyst mimicking the gallbladder. J Clin Ultrasound 14:131, 1986.

Hansen GR, Laing FC: Sonographic evaluation of a left ventricular aneurysm presenting as an upper abdominal mass. J Clin Ultrasound 8:151, 1980.

Jackson FI, Lalani Z: Ultrasound in the diagnosis of lymphoma: A review: J Clin Ultrasound 17:145, 1989.

Khan AN, Bisset RAL: A complex cystic abdominal mass: An unusual presentation of Crohn's disease in an anticoagulated patient. J Clin Ultrasound 16:271, 1988.

Kier R, Chambers SK: Surgical transposition of the ovaries: Imaging findings in 14 patients. AJR 153:1003, 1989.

Kordan B, Payne SD: Fat necrosis simulating a primary tumor of the mesentery: Sonographic diagnosis. J Ultrasound Med 7:345, 1988.

Longmaid HE, Tymkiw J, Rider EA: Sonographic diagnosis of a chylous mesenteric cyst. J Clin Ultrasound 14:458, 1986.

O'Neil JD, Ros PR, Storm BL, et al.: Cystic mesothelioma of the peritoneum. Radiology 170:333, 1989.

Özkan K, Gürses N, Gürses N: Ultrasonic appearance of tuberculous peritonitis. J Clin Ultrasound 15:350, 1987.

Renigers SA, Michael AS, Bardawil WA, et al.: Sonographic findings in leiomyomatosis peritoneales disseminata: A case report and literature review. J Ultrasound Med 4:497, 1985.

Sadola E: Cystic lymphangioma of the jejunal mesentery in an adult. J Clin Ultrasound 15:542, 1987.

Shah IM, King DL: Gray scale sonographic presentation of a mesothelioma of the greater omentum. J Clin Ultrasound 7:147, 1979.

Warhit JM, Fagelman D, Goldman MA, et al.: Ovarian vein thrombophlebitis: Diagnosis by ultrasound and CT. J Clin Ultrasound 12:301, 1984.

Wu CC, Chow KS, Lu TN, et al.: Sonographic features of tuberculous omental cakes in peritoneal tuberculosis. J Clin Ultrasound 16:195, 1988.

FLUID

Common

Ascites
Mesenteric metastases
Peritoneal carcinomatosis
Hematoma
Abscess
After surgery
After peritoneal lavage
Pelvic inflammatory disease (PID)
Ectopic pregnancy

Uncommon

Peritoneal infection
After renal stone removal
    percutaneously
Hepatic tuberculosis
    Hepatic dysfunction
Inferior vena cava (IVC) thrombosis

Brauner M, Buffard MD, Jeantils V, et al.: Sonography and computed tomography of macroscopic tuberculosis of the liver. J Clin Ultrasound 17:563, 1989.
Ivory CM, Dubbins PA, Wells IP, et al.: Ultrasound assessment of local complications of percutaneous renal stone removal. J Clin Ultrasound 17:345, 1989.

RIGHT LOWER QUADRANT CYSTIC STRUCTURE

Common	*Comment*
Appendix in appendicitis	
Normal appendix occasionally	
Ovarian cyst	
Bowel	

Uncommon

Hydrosalpinx	
Meckel's diverticulitis	
Crohn's disease	
Loculated ascites	
Pseudomyxoma peritonei	
Ovarian vein thrombophlebitis	Usually puerperal
Benign mesothelioma, cystic	

Khan AN, Bisset RAL: A complex cystic abdominal mass: An unusual presentation of Crohn's disease in an anticoagulated patient. J Clin Ultrasound 16:271, 1988.

Larson JM, Ellinger DM, Zdybel PJ, et al.: Acute Meckel's diverticulitis: Diagnosis by ultrasonography. J Clin Ultrasound 17:682, 1989.

O'Neil JD, Ros PR, Storm BL, et al.: Cystic mesothelioma of the peritoneum. Radiology 170:333, 1989.

Seale WB: Sonographic findings in a patient with pseudomyxoma peritonei. J Clin Ultrasound 10:441, 1982.

Warhit JM, Fagelman D, Goldman MA, et al.: Ovarian vein thrombophlebitis: Diagnosis by ultrasound and CT. J Clin Ultrasound 12:301, 1984.

Aorta

DISPLACEMENT

                            Comment

Lymphadenopathy
Pancreatic carcinoma
Retroperitoneal fibrosis (rarely)
Inflammatory aneurysm   Hypoechoic area around aorta

Bundy AL, Ritchie WGM: Inflammatory aneurysm of the abdominal aorta. J Clin Ultrasound 12:102, 1984.
Fagan CJ, Larrieu AJ, Amparo EG: Retroperitoneal fibrosis: Ultrasound and CT features. AJR 133:239, 1979.

DILATION

Aneurysm
Simulation by para-aortic sonolucent
    nodes
Incorrect transverse measurement of
    tortuous aorta

PERIAORTIC FLUID

Aortic rupture
Infected aortic prosthetic graft
Retroperitoneal hemorrhage

MASS WITHIN

After umbilical artery catheter in
  neonates
Dissection of aorta
Thrombus within
Sarcoma of aorta

Goodman A, Lipinski JK: Occult thoraco-abdominal dissecting aneurysm in a patient with Marfan's syndrome—diagnosis by real-time ultrasound. J Clin Ultrasound 12:115, 1984.

Seibert JJ, Lindley SG, Corbitt SS, et al.: Clot formation in the renal artery in the neonate demonstrated by ultrasound. J Clin Ultrasound 14:470, 1986.

Inferior Vena Cava

ECHOES WITHIN

Common

Intraluminal clot
Greenfield filter

Uncommon

	Comment
Tumor thrombus	From renal cell carcinoma or hepatocellular carcinoma
Umbrella	
Hydatid disease	
Leiomyosarcoma of IVC	Hypoechoic, heterogeneous
Chiari malformation of right atrium	May prolapse into IVC
Angiomyolipoma of kidney	Echogenic renal mass

Arenson AM, Graham RT, Shaw P, et al.: Angiomyolipoma of the kidney extending into the inferior vena cava: Sonographic and CT findings. AJR 151:1159, 1988.

Bousquet JC, Goze A, Hassan M, et al.: Leiomyosarcoma of the inferior vena cava: Ultrasonographic appearance. J Ultrasound Med 6:7, 1987.

Lewandowski B, Challender J, Dery R: Prolapsing Chiari malformation in tricuspid regurgitation: A moving filling defect in the inferior vena cava. J Ultrasound Med 4:655, 1985.

Morimoto K, Matsui K, Hashimoto T, et al.: Intraatrial extension of hepatocellular carcinoma detected with ultrasound. J Clin Ultrasound 14:466, 1986.

DISPLACEMENT

	Comment
Adrenal masses	
Pancreatic carcinoma	
Renal masses	
Acute pancreatitis	
Leiomyosarcoma of IVC	Fills lumen; hypoechoic, heterogeneous

Bousquet JC, Goze A, Hassan M, et al.: Leiomyosarcoma of the inferior vena cava: Ultrasonographic appearance. J Ultrasound Med 6:7, 1987.

Walls WJ, Templeton JW: The ultrasonic demonstration of inferior vena cava compression: A guide to pancreatic head enlargement with emphasis on neoplasm. Radiology 123:165, 1977.

Wright CH, Maklad F, Rosenthal SJ: Gray-scale ultrasound characteristics of carcinoma of the pancreas. Br J Radiol 52:281, 1979.

Liver

HEPATOMEGALY

Common

Comment

Hepatoma
Metastases
Cirrhosis
Fatty infiltration
Congestive heart failure (CHF)
Infection
  Hepatitis
  Abscess

Uncommon

Lymphoma
Leukemia
Polycythemia vera
Myelofibrosis
Tricuspid insufficiency
Constrictive pericarditis
Budd-Chiari syndrome
Hemochromatosis
Amyloid
Gaucher's disease
Niemann-Pick disease
With adult polycystic kidney disease
  (APKD)
Wolman's disease   Familial

OVERALL INCREASED ECHOGENICITY

Common	Comment
Fatty infiltration	In alcoholics, diabetics; after chemotherapy; after intestinal bypass; see Solid Lesions section
Fibrosis (cirrhosis)	
Chronic hepatitis	
Acute hepatitis	Usually causes no change

Uncommon

Diffuse tuberculosis (TB)
Liver congestion in Budd-Chiari
  syndrome
Diphenylhydantoin toxicity   Can cause liver necrosis
Acquired immunodeficiency syndrome
  (AIDS)
Inappropriate time gain compensation
  (TGC) curve
Glycogen storage disease
Infiltrating malignancy
Liver congestion from CHF
Wilson's disease
Reye's syndrome
Gaucher's disease
Schistosomiasis
Tyrosinemia

Fishman MC, Fischer AH, Arger PH, et al.: Fatal diphenylhydantoin-induced hepatic necrosis: Sonographic-pathologic correlation. J Clin Ultrasound 14:722, 1986.

Giorgio A, Amoroso P, Fico P, et al.: Ultrasound evaluation of uncomplicated and complicated acute viral hepatitis. J Clin Ultrasound 14:675, 1986.

Grumbach K, Coleman BG, Gal AA, et al.: Hepatic and biliary tract abnormalities in patients with AIDS. J Ultrasound Med 8:247, 1989.

Halvorsen R, Korobkin M, Ram P, et al.: CT appearance of focal fatty infiltration of the liver. AJR 139:277, 1982.

Henschke C, Goldman H, Teele R: The hyperechogenic liver in children: Cause and sonographic appearance: AJR 138:841, 1982.

Miller J, Stanley P, Gates G: Radiography of glycogen storage disease. AJR 132:379, 1979.

Nakayama S, Sakata J, Kusumoto S, et al.: Ultrasonic appearance of the liver in hepatic venous outflow obstruction (Budd-Chiari syndrome): A case of pseudohepatic infarct associated with Behçet's disease. J Clin Ultrasound 14:300, 1986.

Scott W, Sanders R, Siegelman S: Irregular fatty infiltration of the liver: Diagnostic dilemmas. AJR 135:67, 1980.

Yee JM, Raghavendra N, Horii SC, et al.: Abdominal sonography in AIDS: A review. J Ultrasound Med 8:705, 1989.

DECREASED ECHOGENICITY

Common

Hepatitis

Uncommon

Lymphoma infiltration
Leukemia infiltration
Amyloid
AIDS

Ginaldi S, Bernardino M, Jing B, et al.: Ultrasonographic patterns of hepatic lymphoma. Radiology 136:427, 1980.
Grumbach K, Coleman BG, Gal AA, et al.: Hepatic and biliary tract abnormalities in patients with AIDS. J Ultrasound Med 8:247, 1989.

BRIGHT PERIPORTAL ECHOES (STARRY-SKY LIVER)

Common

Hepatitis

Comment

Due to decreased echogenicity of adjacent liver

Uncommon

Hepatic Kaposi's sarcoma
Leukemia
Toxic shock syndrome
Burkitt's lymphoma
Oil embolism after lymphangiogram
Cholangitis
Mononucleosis
Cystic fibrosis
Biliary air
Periportal fibrosis
Right heart failure

Giorgio A, Amoroso P, Fico P, et al.: Ultrasound evaluation of uncomplicated and complicated acute viral hepatitis. J Clin Ultrasound 14:675, 1986.
Lee S: Hepatic oil embolism following lymphangiography. J Ultrasound Med 4:357, 1985.
Luburich P, Bru C, Ayuso MC, et al.: Hepatic Kaposi sarcoma in AIDS: US and CT findings. Radiology 175:172, 1990.
Needleman L, Kurtz A, Rifkin M, et al.: Sonography of diffuse benign liver disease: Accuracy of pattern recognition and grading. AJR 146:1011, 1986.
Rak K, Hopper KD, Parker SH: The "starry sky" liver with Burkitt's lymphoma. J Ultrasound Med 7:279, 1988.

INCREASED DIAMETER OF LIVER VESSELS

Common

Right heart failure
Tricuspid insufficiency
CHF

Uncommon

Elevated systemic venous pressure
Hereditary hemorrhagic telangiectasia
  of liver
Tumor within right atrium, IVC, or
  hepatic veins
Budd-Chiari syndrome
Constrictive pericarditis

Goes E, Van Tussenbroeck F, Cottenie F, et al.: Osler's disease diagnosed by ultrasound. J Clin
  Ultrasound 15:129, 1987.

INTRAHEPATIC SHADOWING

Common	Comment
Mucinous carcinoma	
Colon	
Stomach	
Pancreas	
Biliary stones	Occur in Caroli's disease and Oriental cholangiohepatitis
Gallstone	

Uncommon

Gallbladder neck normal	
Previous granulomatous disease	Calcifications
Previous parasitic disease	Calcifications
Neuroblastoma metastasis	
Biliary air	Usually after biliary surgery
Portal venous air	Suggests bowel infarct
Arterial calcification	
Peritoneal carcinomatosis from ovary	Calcifications around liver
Calcifications with biliary cystadenoma or cystadenocarcinoma	
Leprosy	Inhomogeneous echo texture
Biopsy track	

Carvalho P, Allison DJ: Liver biopsy embolization track: Ultrasonic appearance. J Clin Ultrasound 16:426, 1988.

Desai RK, Paushter DM, Armistead J: Intrahepatic arterial calcification mimicking pneumobilia: A potential pitfall in the ultrasound evaluation of biliary tract disease. J Ultrasound Med 8:333, 1989.

Doehring E, Reider F, Dittrich M, et al.: Ultrasonographic findings in the livers of patients with lepromatous leprosy. J Clin Ultrasound 14:179, 1986.

Korobkin M, Stephens DH, Lee JKT, et al.: Biliary cystadenoma and cystadenocarcinoma: CT and sonographic findings. AJR 153:507, 1989.

Pombo F, Lago M, Arrojo L: Letter to Editor re: Ultrasound manifestation of metastatic perihepatic calcifications from ovarian carcinoma. J Clin Ultrasound 17:304, 1989.

Sommer F, Filly R, Minton M: Refractive and reflective acoustic shadowing. AJR 132:973, 1979.

CYSTIC LESIONS, INTRAHEPATIC

Common	Comment
Congenital cysts	May or may not have cysts in kidney
Previous trauma	
Segmental biliary obstruction	Prior surgery, infection, cholangiocarcinoma
With APKD	
Hemangioma	May appear cystic but is really anechoic

Uncommon	
Caroli's disease	Tubular ectasia of biliary tree
Abscesses	
Bacterial	Usually central
Amebic	Usually peripheral with debris
Echinococcal	May be solid or mixed cysts, multiseptated, with daughter cyst
Biliary cystadenoma	
Biliary cystadenocarcinoma	
Cavernous hemangiomas	
Necrotic tumor	Especially metastatic sarcoma
Biloma	
Hepatic foregut cyst	
Choledochal cyst	
Hepatic cystadenoma	
Normal gallbladder	
Pancreatic pseudocyst	May appear to be intrahepatic
Endometrioma	
Posttraumatic biloma	
Tuberculosis	Macrocystic type
Hematoma	
Interposed bowel	
AIDS	
Hypoechoic lesions with septae	Simulate cysts
Mucocele of cystic duct remnant	After transplant
Hepatic artery aneurysm	
Pseudoaneurysm of anastomosis	After transplant

Brauner M, Buffard MD, Jeantils V, et al.: Sonography and computed tomography of macroscopic tuberculosis of the liver. J Clin Ultrasound 17:563, 1989.

Carroll BA: Biliary cystadenoma and cystadenocarcinoma: Gray scale ultrasound appearance. J Clin Ultrasound 6:337, 1978.

Esfahani F, Rooholamini SA, Vessal K: Ultrasonography of hepatic hydatid cysts: New diagnostic signs. J Ultrasound Med 7:443, 1988.

Forrest ME, Cho KJ, Shields JJ, et al.: Biliary cystadenomas: Sonographic-angiographic-pathologic correlations. AJR 135:723, 1980.

Freeny P, Vimont T, Barnett D: Cavernous hemangioma of the liver: Ultrasonography, arteriography, and computed tomography. Radiology 132:143, 1979.

Gould L, Patel A: Ultrasound detection of extrahepatic encapsulated bile: "Biloma." AJR 132:1014, 1979.

Grabb A, Carr L, Goodman JD, et al.: Hepatic endometrioma. J Clin Ultrasound 14:478, 1986.

Harbin WP, Mueller PR, Ferrucci JT, Jr.: Transhepatic cholangiography: Complications and use patterns of the fine-needle technique. Radiology 135:15, 1980.

Kadoya M, Matsui O, Nakanuma Y, et al.: Ciliated hepatic foregut cyst: Radiologic features. Radiology 175:475, 1990.

Kangarloo H, Sarti DA, Sample WF, et al.: Ultrasonographic spectrum of choledochal cysts in children. Pediatr Radiol 9:15, 1980.

Korobkin M, Stephens DH, Lee JKT, et al.: Biliary cystadenoma and cystadenocarcinoma: CT and sonographic findings. AJR 153:507, 1989.

Reuter K, Raptopoulos VD, Cantelmo N, et al.: The diagnosis of a choledochal cyst by ultrasound. Radiology 136:437, 1980.

Roemer C, Ferrucci J, Mueller P, et al.: Hepatic cysts: Diagnosis and therapy by sonographic needle aspiration. AJR 136:1065, 1981.

Schölmerich J, Brigitte AV: Differential diagnosis of anechoic/hypoechoic lesions in the abdomen detected by ultrasound. J Clin Ultrasound 14:339, 1986.

Townsend RR, Laing FC, Jeffrey RB, et al.: Abdominal lymphoma in AIDS: Evaluation with US. Radiology 171:719, 1989.

Weissman HS, Chun KJ, Frank M, et al.: Demonstration of traumatic bile leakage with cholescintigraphy and ultrasonography. AJR 133:843, 1979.

Wiener S, Parulekar S: Scintigraphy and ultrasonography of hepatic hemangioma. Radiology 132:149, 1979.

Wong AD, Pon M, Grymaloski M: An ultrasonic hepatic pseudomass due to colonic interposition. J Clin Ultrasound 16:669, 1988.

Zajko AB, Bennett MJ, Campbell WL, et al.: Mucocele of the cystic duct remnant in eight liver transplant recipients: Findings at cholangiography, CT, and US. Radiology 177:691, 1990.

SOLID LESIONS, INTRAHEPATIC

Common

	Comment
Cavernous hemangioma	Most common benign lesion
Metastases	
Focal nodular hyperplasia	Varying appearance; hyperechoic or hypoechoic
Adenomatous hyperplastic nodules	In cirrhosis
Focal spared areas	Hypoechoic area next to fatty infiltration
Hepatic adenomas	Seen with oral contraceptives, androgens, and Type I glycogen storage disease; hyperechoic or hypoechoic
Focal fatty infiltration	Associated with obesity, alcoholism, diabetes mellitus, pancreatic disease, Wilson's disease, kwashiorkor, intestinal bypass hyperalimentation, pregnancy, Cushing's syndrome, corticosteroids

Uncommon

Capillary hemangioma	Usually echogenic
Abscess	Debris may cause a solid appearance
Amebic abscess	One third are unifocal; may have through transmission
Bile duct hamartomas	
Fungal abscess	Usually immunosuppressed patients
Hepatoma	May be hyperechogenic or hypoechogenic; look for portal venous invasion
Extramedullary hematopoiesis	
Candidiasis	May be hypoechoic, hyperechoic, or bull's eye
Decreased portal flow	Leads to focal spared area; is hypoechoic
Echinococcus (hydatid) cysts	
Granuloma from visceral larva migrans	Multiple; hypoechoic areas
Cholangiocarcinoma	May be intraluminal or exophytic
Lymphoma	Usually infiltrative, not focal; occurs in patients taking cyclosporine
Tuberculosis	
Leprosy	
Wound abscess mimicking liver lesion	

SOLID LESIONS, INTRAHEPATIC (Continued)

Uncommon (Continued)	Comment
Hepatic artery aneurysm	Hypoechoic center
Diphenylhydantoin toxicity	Can cause areas of necrosis
Regenerating cirrhotic nodules	
Angiomyolipomas	Echogenic
Erythromycin-induced hepatitis	Echogenic masses
Hepatic Kaposi's sarcoma	Hyperechoic nodules
AIDS	Focal masses in 19%
Fat in hepatocellular carcinoma	Echogenic area
Multifocal cytomegalovirus (CMV) or AIDS	From fatty infiltration
Hematoma	
Lipoma	

Abbitt PL, Teates CD: The sonographic appearance of extramedullary hematopoiesis in the liver. J Clin Ultrasound 17:280, 1989.

Arai K, Matsui O, Takashima T, et al.: Focal spared areas in fatty liver caused by regional decreased portal flow. AJR 151:300, 1988.

Berry M, Bazaz R, Bhargava S: Amebic liver abscess: Sonographic diagnosis and management. J Clin Ultrasound 14:239, 1986.

Brandt DJ, Johnson CD, Stephens DH, et al.: Imaging of fibrolamellar hepatocellular carcinoma. AJR 151:295, 1988.

Cottone M, Marceno M, Maringhini A, et al.: Ultrasound in the diagnosis of hepatocellular carcinoma associated with cirrhosis. Radiology 147:517, 1983.

Doehring E, Reider F, Dittrich M, et al.: Ultrasonographic findings in the livers of patients with lepromatous leprosy. J Clin Ultrasound 14:179, 1986.

Esfahani F, Rooholamini SA, Vessal K: Ultrasonography of hepatic hydatid cysts: New diagnostic signs. J Ultrasound Med 7:443, 1988.

Fishman MC, Fischer AH, Arger PH: Fatal diphenylhydantoin-induced hepatic necrosis: Sonographic-pathologic correlation. J Clin Ultrasound 14:722, 1986.

Garcia FJ, Marti-Bonmati L, Menor F, et al.: Echogenic forms of hydatid cysts: Sonographic diagnosis. J Clin Ultrasound 16:305, 1988.

Grossman H, Ram P, Coleman R, et al.: Hepatic ultrasonography in Type I glycogen storage disease (von Gierke's disease). Radiology 141:753, 1981.

Grumbach K, Coleman BG, Gal AA, et al.: Hepatic and biliary tract abnormalities in patients with AIDS. J Ultrasound Med 8:247, 1989.

Hirata T, Yamasaki K, Li YG, et al.: Demonstration of hepatic granuloma due to visceral larva migrans by ultrasonography. J Clin Ultrasound 18:429, 1990.

Honda H, Franken EA, Jr., Barloon TJ, et al.: Hepatic lymphoma in cyclosporine-treated transplant recipients: Sonographic and CT findings. AJR 152:501, 1989.

King DJ, Bayliss AP, Bennett B, et al.: Unusual presentation of opportunistic infections in patients with leukemia:Identification of fungal lesions by ultrasound. J Clin Ultrasound 15:486, 1987.

Livraghi T, Gangalli G, Bettori C: Adenomatous hyperplastic nodules in the cirrhotic liver: A therapeutic approach. Work in Progress. Radiology 170:155, 1989.

Luburich P, Bru C, Ayuso MC, et al.: Hepatic Kaposi sarcoma in AIDS: US and CT findings. Radiology 175:172, 1990.

Nelson RC, Chezmar JL: Diagnostic approach to hepatic hemangiomas. Radiology 176:11, 1990.

Nesbit GM, Johnson CD, James EM, et al.: Cholangiocarcinoma: Diagnosis and evaluation of resectability by CT and sonography as procedures complementary to cholangiography. AJR 151:933, 1988.

Pastakia B, Shawker TH, Thaler M, et al.: Hepatosplenic candidiasis: Wheels within wheels. Radiology 166:417, 1988.

Pulpeiro JR, Orduna M, Jimenez J, et al.: Primary hepatocellular adenoma in men. J Clin Ultrasound 17:269, 1989.

Rigauts HD, Selleslag DL, Van Eyken PL, et al.: Erythromycin-induced hepatitis: Simulator of malignancy. Radiology 169:661, 1988.

Robinson D, Grant EG, Haller JO, et al.: Hepatic angiomyolipomas in tuberous sclerosis: Report of two cases. J Ultrasound Med 8:575, 1989.

Scatarige J, Fishman E, Sanders R: The sonographic "scar sign" in focal nodular hyperplasia of the liver. J Ultrasound Med 1:275, 1982.

Shawker TH, Hill M, Hill S, et al.: Ultrasound appearance of extramedullary hematopoiesis. J Ultrasound Med 6:283, 1987.

Tan A, Shen JF, Hecht AH: Sonogram of multiple bile duct hamartomas. J Clin Ultrasound 17:667, 1989.

Townsend RR, Laing FC, Jeffrey RB, et al.: Abdominal lymphoma in AIDS: Evaluation with US. Radiology 171:719, 1989.

Vieco PT, Rochon L, Lisbona A: Multifocal cytomegalovirus-associated hepatic lesions simulating metastases in AIDS. Radiology 176:123, 1990.

Wang SS, Chiang JH, Tsai YT, et al.: Focal hepatic fatty infiltration as a cause of pseudotumors: Ultrasonographic patterns and clinical differentiation. J Clin Ultrasound 18:401, 1990.

Yiengpruksawan A, Pow-Anpongkul S, Ganepola GAP, et al.: Echogenic wound abscess mimicking hepatic mass on ultrasonography. J Clin Ultrasound 14:376, 1986.

Yoshikawa J, Matsui O, Takashima T, et al.: Fatty metamorphosis in hepatocellular carcinoma: Radiologic features in 10 cases. AJR 151:717, 1988.

CALCIFICATIONS IN FOCAL HEPATIC LESION

Common	Comment

Hemangioma, cavernous
Metastatic adenocarcinoma
    Colon
    Stomach
    Rectum
    Pancreas
    Thyroid
    Lung carcinoma
    Ovarian carcinoma
    Renal cell carcinoma
    Hepatocellular carcinoma
Calcified gallbladder

Uncommon

TB
Teratoma
Echinococcus
Biliary cystadenoma or
   cystadenocarcinoma
Abscess   Especially from ameba

Barnett PH, Zerhouni EA, White RJ, Jr., et al.: Computed tomography in the diagnosis of cavernous hemangioma of the liver. AJR 134:439, 1987.

Esfahani F, Rooholamini SA, Vessal K: Ultrasonography of hepatic hydatid cysts: New diagnostic signs. J Ultrasound Med 7:433, 1988.

Garcia FJ, Marti-Bonmati L, Menor F, et al.: Echogenic forms of hydatid cysts: Sonographic diagnosis. J Clin Ultrasound 16:305, 1988.

Korobkin M, Stephens DH, Lee JKT, et al.: Biliary cystadenoma and cystadenocarcinoma: CT and sonographic findings. AJR 153:507, 1989.

Kraudel K, Williams CH: Ultrasound case report of hepatic teratoma in newborn. J Clin Ultrasound 12:98, 1984.

Nelson RC, Chezmar JL: Diagnostic approach to hepatic hemangiomas. Radiology 176:11, 1990.

INTRAHEPATIC CALCIFICATIONS
(NO ACCOMPANYING LESION)

Common   *Comment*

Granuloma
Biliary stone   Look for dilated duct

Uncommon

Calcified prior abscess
Calcified prior hematoma
Calcified parasite
Leprosy   Inhomogeneous echo texture
Echinococcus

Doehring E, Reider F, Dittrich M, et al.: Ultrasonographic findings in the livers of patients with lepromatous leprosy. J Clin Ultrasound 14:179, 1986.
Garcia FJ, Marti-Bonmati L, Menor F, et al.: Echogenic forms of hydatid cysts: Sonographic diagnosis. J Clin Ultrasound 16:305, 1988.

INVASION OF HEPATIC VESSELS BY A MASS

Common

Hepatocellular carcinoma

Uncommon

Metastases
Lymphoma

LESION WITH ECHOGENIC RIM

Common

Hydatid disease
Amebic abscess
Hepatoma

Garcia FJ, Marti-Bonmati L, Menor F, et al.: Echogenic forms of hydatid cysts: Sonographic diagnosis. J Clin Ultrasound 16:305, 1988.
Hussain S: Diagnostic criteria of hydatid disease on hepatic sonography. J Ultrasound Med 4:603, 1985.

Gallbladder

SEPTAE

	Comment
Phrygian cap	Near fundus
Hartmann's pouch	Near neck
Mucosal sloughing in acute cholecystitis	

Cheong LL, Khan AN, Armstrong GR: Ultrasonic demonstration of an intraluminal pseudomembrane in the gallbladder: A definitive sign of acute cholecystitis? J Clin Ultrasound 17:449, 1989.

COURVOISIER GALLBLADDER (OVERDISTENDED)

	Comment
Biliary obstruction	
Large but normal	
Cystic duct obstruction in cholecystitis	Acute or chronic
Acalculous cholecystitis	
Typhoid fever	

Cohen EK, Stringer DA, Smith CR: Hydrops of the gallbladder in typhoid fever as demonstrated by sonography. J Clin Ultrasound 14:633, 1986.

ECHOES WITHIN

Common

Stones
Sludge

Comment

Occurs with biliary stasis; may occur
    with cystic duct obstruction

Uncommon

Fold in gallbladder
Acute cholecystitis

Hemobilia
Empyema
Stone fragments after extracorporeal
  shock wave lithotripsy (ESWL)
Polyps, adenomatous or inflammatory

AIDS
Carcinoma

Hemorrhagic cholecystitis
Sarcoma of gallbladder
Metastases
Emphysematous cholecystitis
Milk of calcium
Clonorchiasis
Pus
Papilloma
Epithelial cyst
Ectopic pancreas
Ectopic gastric mucosa
Feces after fistula formation

Sloughing of wall may produce
    membrane within gallbladder

Pus may produce echoes

Not affected by changes in patient
    position
Due to sludge
Thickening of wall or complex
    echogenic mass

Echogenic mass
Usually melanoma
Gas produces echoes

Worms in gallbladder, nonshadowing

Bloom RA, Libson E, Lebensart PD, et al.: The ultrasound spectrum of emphysematous cholecystitis.
  J Clin Ultrasound 17:251, 1989.
Carter SJ, Rutledge J, Hirsch JH, et al.: Papillary adenoma of the gallbladder. Ultrasonic demonstration.
  J Clin Ultrasound 6:433, 1978.

Cheong LL, Khan AN, Armstrong GR: Ultrasonic demonstration of an intraluminal pseudomembrane in the gallbladder: A definitive sign of acute cholecystitis? J Clin Ultrasound 17:449, 1989.

Childress MH: Sonographic features of milk of calcium cholecystitis. J Clin Ultrasound 14:312, 1986.

Chinn DH, Miller EI, Piper N: Hemorrhagic cholecystitis: Sonographic appearance and clinical presentation. J Ultrasound Med 6:313, 1987.

Coelho JCU, Wallbach A, Kasting G, et al.: Ultrasonic diagnosis of primary sarcoma of the gallbladder. J Clin Ultrasound 12:168, 1984.

Conrad MR, Janes JO, Dietchy J: Significance of low-level echoes within the gallbladder. AJR 2:967, 1979.

Dyer R, Montgomery J, Thiele A, et al.: Right upper quadrant renal milk of calcium mimicking limy bile. J Clin Ultrasound 15:140, 1987.

Filly RA, Allen B, Minton MJ, et al.: In vitro investigation of the origin of echoes within biliary sludge. J Clin Ultrasound 8:193, 1980.

Grant EG, Smirniotopoulos JG: Intraluminal gallbladder hematoma: Sonographic evidence of hemobilia. J Clin Ultrasound 11:507, 1983.

Grumbach K, Coleman BG, Gal AA, et al.: Hepatic and biliary tract abnormalities in patients with AIDS. J Ultrasound Med 8:247, 1989.

Kane RA: Ultrasonographic diagnosis of gangrenous cholecystitis and empyema of the gallbladder. Radiology 134:191, 1980.

Khouri MR, Goldszmidt JB, Laufer I, et al.: Intact stones or fragments? Potential pitfalls in the imaging of patients after biliary extracorporeal shock wave lithotripsy. Radiology 177:147, 1990.

Kumar A, Aggarwal S, Berry M, et al.: Ultrasonography of carcinoma of the gallbladder: An analysis of 80 cases. J Clin Ultrasound 18:715, 1990.

Kuo YC, Liu JY, Sheen IS, et al.: Ultrasonographic difficulties and pitfalls in diagnosing primary carcinoma of the gallbladder. J Clin Ultrasound 18:639, 1990.

Lim JH, Ko YT, Lee DH, et al.: Clonorchiasis: Sonographic findings in 59 proved cases. AJR 152:761, 1989.

Sax SL, Athey PA, Lamki N, et al.: Sonographic findings in traumatic hemobilia: Report of two cases and review of the literature. J Clin Ultrasound 16:29, 1988.

Thurber LA, Cooperberg PL, Clement JG, et al.: Echogenic fluid: A pitfall in the ultrasonographic diagnosis of cystic lesions. J Clin Ultrasound 7:273, 1979.

SHADOWS FROM WALL

Comment

Emphysematous cholecystitis
Porcelain gallbladder
Multiple stones

Especially in Rokitansky-Aschoff sinuses

Gas in duodenum behind gallbladder
Refraction from edge of gallbladder

Bloom RA, Libson E, Lebensart PD, et al.: The ultrasound spectrum of emphysematous cholecystitis. J Clin Ultrasound 17:251, 1989.

Hunter ND, Macintosh PK: Acute emphysematous cholecystitis: An ultrasonic diagnosis. AJR 134:592, 1980.

MacDonald FR, Cooperberg PL, Cohen MM: The WES triad. A specific sonographic sign of gallstones in the contract gallbladder. Gastrointest Radiol 6:39, 1981.

NONVISUALIZATION

Common	*Comment*
Prior cholecystectomy	
Calcification of near wall causing nonrecognition	

Uncommon

Agenesis of gallbladder	Incidence of .04%
Ectopic gallbladder	
Anomalous shape of gallbladder	
Gallbladder contracted or empty	
Severe hepatic dysfunction	
Biliary obstruction proximal to cystic duct	
Microgallbladder	Seen in cystic fibrosis
Shadowing from emphysematous cholecystitis	
Sludge in gallbladder causing gallbladder to resemble liver	
Situs inversus	
Compression by adjacent mass	

Blanton DE, Bream CA, Mandel SR: Gallbladder ectopia: A review of anomalies of position. Am J Radiol 121:396, 1974.

Greaves FW, Nguyen KT, Sauerbrei EE: Retrohepatic gallbladder diagnosed by sonography and scintigraphy. J Can Assoc Radiol 34:319, 1983.

Hammond DI: Unusual causes of sonographic nonvisualization or nonrecognition of the gallbladder: A review. J Clin Ultrasound 16:77, 1988.

Reining JW, Stanley JH: Sonographic hepatization of the gallbladder: A cause of nonvisualization of the gallbladder by cholecystosonography. J Clin Ultrasound 12:234, 1984.

Taybi H: The biliary tract in children, in Margulis AR, Burhenne HJ (eds): *Alimentary Tract Roentgenology*, Vol 2. St. Louis, CV Mosby, 1973, p 1504.

Youngwirth LD, Peters JC, Perry MC: The suprahepatic gallbladder. Radiology 149:57, 1983.

WALL THICKENING

Common	Comment
Gallbladder wall fold	
Acute cholecystitis	
Chronic cholecystitis	
Hepatic dysfunction	
CHF	
Hepatitis	
Partial contraction after eating	
Tumefacient sludge	

Uncommon

Polyps	Adenomatous or cholesterol
Carcinoma of gallbladder	
Metastasis	Usually melanoma
Adenomyomatosis of gallbladder	
Renal disease	
Sepsis	
Alcoholic hepatitis	
Hypoalbuminemia	
Ascites	
Papillary adenomas	
Biliary pus	
Biliary clot	
Gallbladder torsion	
Varices	
Cirrhosis	
Chronic renal failure	
Acute pyelonephritis	
Mononucleosis	
Primary sclerosing cholangitis	Associated with ulcerative colitis
Hemobilia	May get submucosal hematoma after trauma

AIDS
Hemorrhagic cholecystitis
Xanthogranulomatous cholecystitis

Brandt DJ, MacCarty RL, Charboneau JW, et al.: Gallbladder disease in patients with primary sclerosing cholangitis. AJR 150:571, 1988.

Carter SJ, Rutledge J, Hirsch JH, et al.: Papillary adenoma of the gallbladder: Ultrasonic demonstration. J Clin Ultrasound 6:433, 1978.

Chinn DH, Miller EI, Piper N: Hemorrhagic cholecystitis: Sonographic appearance and clinical presentation. J Ultrasound Med 6:313, 1987.

Costa-Greco MA: Adenomyomatosis of the gallbladder. J Clin Ultrasound 15:198, 1987.

Grumbach K, Coleman BG, Gal AA, et al.: Hepatic and biliary tract abnormalities in patients with AIDS. J Ultrasound Med 8:247, 1989.

Hammond DI, MacLean RS: Gallbladder wall thickening in an elderly woman with infectious mononucleosis. J Clin Ultrasound 15:558, 1987.

Kumar L, Aggarwal S, Berry M, et al.: Ultrasonography of carcinoma of the gallbladder: An analysis of 80 cases. J Clin Ultrasound 18:715, 1990.

Kuo YC, Liu JY, Sheen IS, et al.: Ultrasonographic difficulties and pitfalls in diagnosing primary carcinoma of the gallbladder. J Clin Ultrasound 18:639, 1990.

Laing FC, Federle MP, Jeffrey RB, et al.: Ultrasonic evaluation of patients with acute right upper quadrant pain. Radiology 140:449, 1981.

Lichtman JB, Varma VA: Ultrasound demonstration of xanthogranulomatous cholecystitis. J Clin Ultrasound 15:342, 1987.

Ralls PW, Mayekawa DS, Lee KP, et al.: Gallbladder wall varices: Diagnosis with color flow Doppler sonography. J Clin Ultrasound 16:595, 1988.

Ralls PW, Quinn MF, Juttner HU, et al.: Gallbladder wall thickening: Patients without intrinsic gallbladder disease. AJR 137:65, 1981.

Rice J, Sauerbrei EE, Semogas P, et al.: The sonographic appearance of adenomyomatosis of the gallbladder. J Clin Ultrasound 9:336, 1981.

Romano AJ, vanSonnenberg E, Casola G, et al.: Gallbladder and bile duct abnormalities in AIDS: Sonographic findings in eight patients. AJR 150:123, 1988.

Saigh J, Williams S, Cawley K, et al.: Varices: A cause of focal gallbladder wall thickening. J Ultrasound Med 4:371, 1985.

Sanders RC: The significance of sonographic gallbladder wall thickening. J Clin Ultrasound 8:143, 1980.

Sax SL, Athey PA, Lamki N, et al.: Sonographic findings in traumatic hemobilia: Report of two cases and review of the literature. J Clin Ultrasound 16:29, 1988.

Shlaer WJ, Leopold GR, Scheible FW: Sonography of the thickened gallbladder wall: A nonspecific finding. AJR 136:337, 1981.

Talarico HP, Rubens D: Gallbladder wall thickening in acute pyelonephritis. J Clin Ultrasound 18:653, 1990.

Wegener M, Börsch G, Schneider J, et al.: Gallbladder wall thickening: A frequent finding in various nonbiliary disorders—A prospective ultrasonographic study. J Clin Ultrasound 15:307, 1987.

Worthen NJ, Uszler JM, Funamura JL: Cholecystitis: Prospective evaluation of sonography and ^{99m}Tc-HIDA cholescintigraphy. AJR 137:973, 1981.

Ye, HC, Weiss MF, Gerson CD: Torsion of the gallbladder: The ultrasonographic features. J Clin Ultrasound 17:123, 1989.

PERICHOLECYSTIC FLUID

Common	Comment
Acute cholecystitis with or without perforation	
Ascites	

Uncommon

Associated with pancreatitis	
Associated with peptic ulcer disease	Fluid extends along hepatoduodenal ligament
Gallbladder torsion	
After perforated appendix	
Pericholecystic abscess	
Hematoma	
AIDS	

Chau WK, Na AT, Feng TT, et al.: Ultrasound diagnosis of perforation of the gallbladder: Real-time application and the demonstration of a new sonographic sign. J Clin Ultrasound 16:358, 1988.

Evans RH, Colbert RF: Acute perforated appendicitis—An unusual variant simulating acute acalculous cholecystitis. J Clin Ultrasound 16:513, 1988.

Nyberg DA, Laing FC: Ultrasonographic findings in peptic ulcer disease and pancreatitis that simulate primary gallbladder disease. J Ultrasound Med 2:303, 1983.

Yeh HC, Weiss MF, Gerson CD: Torsion of the gallbladder: The ultrasonographic features. J Clin Ultrasound 17:123, 1989.

CYSTS WITHIN THE WALL

	Comment
Rokitansky-Aschoff sinuses	Communication with gallbladder lumen
Luschka's crypts	No communication with gallbladder lumen
Diverticulae	
Mesothelial cysts	
Xanthogranulomatous cholecystitis	Hypoechoic nodules within wall
Varices of wall	

Costa-Greco, MA: Adenomyomatosis of the gallbladder. J Clin Ultrasound 15:198, 1987.

Hoffman CJ, Hales ED, Malachowski ME, et al.: Mesothelial cyst of the gallbladder. J Clin Ultrasound 17:50, 1989.

Lichtman JB, Varma VA: Ultrasound demonstration of xanthogranulomatous cholecystitis. J Clin Ultrasound 15:342, 1987.

Ralls PW, Mayekawa DS, Lee KP, et al.: Gallbladder wall varices: Diagnosis with color flow Doppler sonography. J Clin Ultrasound 16:595, 1988.

Biliary System

"TOO MANY TUBES" IN THE LIVER

	Comment
Dilated intrahepatic bile ducts	
Biliary obstruction	
Caroli's disease	
Dilated intrahepatic arteries	With cirrhosis and portal hypertension
Angiodysplasia of hepatic artery	Reported in hereditary hemorrhagic telangiectasia syndrome

Choi BI, Yeon KM, Kim SH, et al.: Caroli disease: Central dot sign in CT. Radiology 174:161, 1990.

Goes E, Van Tussenbroeck F, Cottenie F, et al.: Osler's disease diagnosed by ultrasound. J Clin Ultrasound 15:129, 1987.

Wing VW, Laing FC, Jeffrey RB, et al.: Sonographic differentiation of enlarged hepatic arteries from dilated intrahepatic bile ducts. AJR 145:57, 1985.

ENLARGED COMMON DUCT

Common	*Comment*
Bile duct obstruction	
Biliary stone	
Pancreatic carcinoma	
Cholangiocarcinoma	Intraluminal or exophytic
Ampullary carcinoma	
Lymphoma of pancreas	
Papilloma of common duct	
Choledochal cyst	
Biliary clonorchiasis	Worms may move
AIDS	Usually extrahepatic enlargement only
Clonorchiasis	Intrahepatic ducts dilated; extrahepatic may be normal
Recurrent pyogenic cholangitis	

Cardoza J, Schrumpf J, Skioldebrand C, et al.: Biliary obstruction caused by a papilloma of the common hepatic duct. J Ultrasound Med 7:467, 1988.

Chan F-L, Man S-W, Leong LLY, et al.: Evaluation of recurrent pyogenic cholangitis with CT: Analysis of 50 patients. Radiology 170:165, 1989.

Grumbach K, Coleman BG, Gal AA, et al.: Hepatic and biliary tract abnormalities in patients with AIDS. J Ultrasound Med 8:247, 1989.

Lim JH, Ko YT, Lee DH, et al.: Clonorchiasis: Sonographic findings in 59 proved cases. AJR 152:761, 1989.

Morikawa P, Ishida H, Niizawa M, et al.: Sonographic features of biliary clonorchiasis. J Clin Ultrasound 16:655, 1988.

Nesbit GM, Johnson CD, James EM, et al.: Cholangiocarcinoma: Diagnosis and evaluation of resectability by CT and sonography as procedures complementary to cholangiography. AJR 151:933, 1988.

Romano AJ, vanSonnenberg E, Casola G, et al.: Gallbladder and bile duct abnormalities in AIDS: Sonographic findings in eight patients. AJR 150:123, 1988.

Swartz TR, Ritchie WGM: Bile duct obstruction secondary to lymphomatous involvement of the pancreas. J Clin Ultrasound 11:391, 1983.

ECHOES WITHIN THE COMMON DUCT

Common	*Comment*
Sludge	Especially seen in obstructed duct

Uncommon	
Pus	Usually obstructed system
Clonorchiasis	Worms may move
Hemobilia	
Pneumobilia	
Recurrent pyogenic cholangitis	Also know as primary cholangitis or Oriental cholangitis
Cholangiocarcinoma	
Feces	From biliary-enteric fistula
Hepatoma	

Allen KS, Lebensart PD, Arger PH, et al.: Sonographic demonstration of echogenic hemobilia. J Clin Ultrasound 16:681, 1988.

Chan F-L, Man S-W, Leong LLY, et al.: Evaluation of recurrent pyogenic cholangitis with CT: Analysis of 50 patients. Radiology 170:165, 1989.

McSherry CK, Stubenbord WT, Glenn F: The significance of air in the biliary system and liver. Surg Gynecol Obstet 128:49, 1969.

Morikawa P, Ishida H, Niizawa M, et al.: Sonographic features of biliary clonorchiasis. J Clin Ultrasound 16:655, 1988.

Skaane P: Ultrasonic demonstration of a pedunculated colonic polyp. J Clin Ultrasound 15:204, 1987.

ECHOGENIC BILE DUCT WALL

Common

Relatively hypoechoic liver

Uncommon

Sclerosing cholangitis
Clonorchiasis

Lim JH, Ko YT, Lee DH, et al.: Clonorchiasis: Sonographic findings in 59 proved cases. AJR 152:761, 1989.

Pancreas

FOCAL MASS

Common	Comment
Carcinoma	
Lymphomatous nodes	
Pseudocyst	
Pancreatitis, especially acute	

Uncommon

Metastatic nodes	
Cystadenoma	Mainly hypoechoic
Cystadenocarcinoma	
Islet cell tumor	
Pancreatic phlegmon	
Congenital cysts	In association with polycystic kidney disease
Retention cysts	Due to prior duct obstruction
Abscess	
Peripancreatic adenopathy	
Sarcoidosis	
Lipomatosis of pancreas	Hypoechoic

Bock E, Grandinetti F, Corcioni E, et al.: Lipomatosis of the pancreas: Mistake in diagnostic imaging. J Clin Ultrasound 14:398, 1986.
Sagalow BR, Miller CL, Wechsler RJ: Pancreatic sarcoidosis mimicking pancreatic cancer. J Clin Ultrasound 16:131, 1988.

CYSTIC LESIONS

Common	Comment
Pseudocyst	May have debris

Uncommon

Posttraumatic cysts	
Cystadenoma	Cysts ≤2 cm means microcystic; >2 cm means mucinous
Cystic adenocarcinoma	
Islet cell tumors	Anechoic; not usually cystic
Abscess	
Duodenal cyst	
Dilated distal common bile duct	
Congenital cysts	
Hematoma	
Lymphoma	May simulate cyst

Fried AM, Pulmano CM, Mostowycz L: Duodenal duplication cyst: Sonographic and angiographic features. Am J Roentgenol 128:863, 1977.

Johnson CD, Stephens DH, Charboneau JW, et al.: Cystic pancreatic tumors: CT and sonographic assessment. AJR 151:1133, 1988.

Schölmerich J, Volk BA: Differential diagnosis of anechoic/hypoechoic lesions in the abdomen detected by ultrasound. J Clin Ultrasound 14:339, 1986.

DIFFUSELY INCREASED SIZE

	Comment
Acute pancreatitis	May be focal also
Pancreatic phlegmon	
Chronic pancreatitis	May be focal

ECHOGENIC

Common	*Comment*
Chronic pancreatitis	

Uncommon

Cystic fibrosis	Fatty infiltration
Obese patients	Fatty infiltration
Diabetes	Fatty infiltration
Steroid ingestion	

Gupta AK, Arenson AM, McKee JD: Effect of steroid ingestion on pancreatic echogenicity. J Clin Ultrasound 15:171, 1987.

HYPOECHOIC

Acute pancreatitis
Lymphoma of pancreas

Jackson FI, Lalani Z: Ultrasound in the diagnosis of lymphoma: A review. J Clin Ultrasound 17:145, 1989.

DECREASED SIZE

Chronic pancreatitis
Cystic fibrosis

PERIPANCREATIC HYPOECHOIC MASSES

Common

Pseudocyst
Fluid-filled bowel

Uncommon

Aneurysm of hepatic or splenic arteries
Loculated ascites
Dilated vein
Lymphoma

CALCIFICATIONS

Common	**Comment**
Chronic pancreatitis	
Pseudocysts	

Uncommon	
Gallstone pancreatitis	Does not usually calcify
Carcinoma of pancreas	Does not usually calcify
Hyperparathyroidism	
Cystic fibrosis	Late finding
Kwashiorkor	
Hereditary pancreatitis	
Cystadenomas	
Cystadenocarcinomas	

Spleen

ENLARGED

Common	Comment
Lymphoma	
Portal hypertension	
Mononucleosis	
Leukemia	

Uncommon

	Comment
AIDS	
Metastasis	
Gaucher's disease	
Acute splenic sequestration crisis	In sickle cell disease
Leukemia	Especially chronic myelocytic leukemia (CML)
Multiple myeloma	
Wilson's disease	
Myelofibrosis	
Malaria	
Reticulum cell sarcoma	
Kala-azar	
Still's disease	
Glycogen storage diseases	
Hereditary spherocytosis	
Hepatitis	
Hemangioma or hemangiosarcoma	
Septicemia	
Sickle cell disease	
Brucellosis	
Hemolysis	
Typhoid	
TB	
Typhus	
Histoplasmosis	
Sarcoid	
Amyloid	
Rheumatoid arthritis	Felty's syndrome
Lupus	
Wolman's disease	

Goerg C, Schwerk WB, Goerg K, et al.: Sonographic patterns of the affected spleen in malignant lymphoma. J Clin Ultrasound 18:569, 1990.

Ishibashi H, Okumura Y, Higuchi N, et al.: Differentiation of mononucleosis from hepatitis by sonographic measurement of spleen size. J Clin Ultrasound 15:313, 1987.

Roshkow JE, Sanders LM: Acute splenic sequestration crisis in two adults with sickle cell disease: US, CT, and MR imaging findings. Radiology 177:723, 1990.

Schoenfeld A, Tepper R, Stein L, et al.: Ultrasonographic aspects of Gaucher's disease: Report of a patient during three pregnancies. J Clin Ultrasound 15:207, 1987.

Stevens PG, Kumari-Subaiya SS, Kahn LB: Splenic involvement in Gaucher's disease: Sonographic findings. J Clin Ultrasound 15:397, 1987.

Yee JM, Raghavendra BN, Horii SC, et al.: Abdominal sonography in AIDS: A review. J Ultrasound Med 8:705, 1989.

FOCAL ABNORMALITIES

Common

	Comment
Abscess	Cystic or complex
Prior granulomatous disease	Calcifications
Cysts	Congenital or posttraumatic
Metastases	Melanoma most common
Infarct	Wedge-shaped; hypoechoic early, echogenic late
Hematoma	
Infarction	

Uncommon

Candida or fungus	May present as target lesion; hypoechoic lesion
Lymphoma	Usually infiltrative and nonfocal in adults; two thirds will have large spleen
Hemangioma	
TB	If active, may have defects
Cat-scratch fever	
Left lobe of liver mimicking fluid collection	
Hydatid disease	
Extramedullary hematopoiesis	Hypoechoic
Gaucher's disease	
Splenic sequestration crisis	Sickle cell disease

Brauner M, Buffard MD, Jeantils V, et al.: Sonography and computed tomography of macroscopic tuberculosis of the liver. J Clin Ultrasound 17:563, 1989.

Costeno P, Kane RA, Oster J, et al.: Focal splenic disease demonstrated by ultrasound and computerized tomography. J Can Assoc Radiol 36:22, 1983.

Crivello MS, Peterson IM, Austin RM: Left lobe of the liver mimicking perisplenic collections. J Clin Ultrasound 14:697, 1986.

Goerg C, Schwerk WB: Splenic infarction: Sonographic patterns, diagnosis, follow-up, and complications. Radiology 174:803, 1990.

Goerg C, Schwerk WB, Goerg K, et al.: Sonographic patterns of the affected spleen in malignant lymphoma. J Clin Ultrasound 18:569, 1990.

Gupta RK, Pant CS, Ganguly SK: Ultrasound demonstration of amebic splenic abscess. J Clin Ultrasound 15:555, 1987.

Jackson FI, Lalani Z: Ultrasound in the diagnosis of lymphoma: A review. J Clin Ultrasound 17:145, 1989.

Maresca G, Mirk P, De Gaetano AM, et al.: Sonographic patterns in splenic infarct. J Clin Ultrasound 14:23, 1986.

Pastakie B, Shawker TH, Thaler M, et al.: Hepatosplenic candidiasis: Wheels within wheels. Radiology 166:417, 1988.

Roshkow JE, Sanders LM: Acute splenic sequestration crisis in two adults with sickle cell disease: US, CT, and MR imaging findings. Radiology 177:723, 1990.

Shawker TH, Hill M, Hill S, et al.: Ultrasound appearance of extramedullary hematopoiesis. J Ultrasound Med 6:283, 1987.

Shirkhoda A, Wallace S, Sokhandan M: Computerized tomography and ultrasonography in splenic infarction. J Can Assoc Radiol 36:29, 1985.

Solbiati L, Bossi MC, Bellotti E, et al.: Focal lesions in the spleen: Sonographic patterns and guided biopsy. Am J Roentgenol 140:59, 1983.

Stevens PG, Kumari-Subaiya SS, Kahn LB: Splenic involvement in Gaucher's disease: Sonographic findings. J Clin Ultrasound 15:397, 1987.

Stutte H, Müller PH, d'Hoedt B, et al.: Ultrasonographic diagnosis of melanoma metastases in liver, gallbladder, and spleen. J Ultrasound Med 8:541, 1989.

CYSTS

Common	*Comment*
Congenital	Epithelial lining
Posttraumatic cyst	

Uncommon

Parasitic	
Neoplastic	
Lymphangiomas	
Cavernous hemangiomas	
Abscess	
Hematoma	
Capillary hemangioma	
Epidermoid cyst	
Hamartoma	May appear cystic or anechoic
Rupture with fissure	May simulate cyst
Hydatid disease	
Splenic sequestration crisis	Sickle cell disease

Bhimji SD, Cooperberg PL, Naiman S, et al.: Ultrasound diagnosis of splenic cysts. Radiology 122:787, 1977.

Blank E, Campbell JR: Epidermoid cysts of the spleen. Pediatrics 51:75, 1973.

Brinkley AA, Lee JKT: Cystic hamartoma of the spleen: CT and sonographic findings. J Clin Ultrasound 9:136, 1981.

Dembner AG, Taylor KJW: Gray scale sonographic diagnosis: Multiple congenital splenic cysts. J Clin Ultrasound 6:143, 1978.

Fowler RH: Cystic tumors of the spleen. Int Abst Surg 70:213, 1940.

Goldfinger M, Cohen MM, Steinhardt MI, et al.: Sonography and percutaneous aspiration of splenic epidermoid cyst. J Clin Ultrasound 14:147, 1986.

Kaufman RA, Silver TM, Wesley JR: Preoperative diagnosis of splenic cysts in children by gray scale ultrasonography. J Pediatr Surg 14:450, 1979.

Manor A, Starinsky R, Garfinkel D, et al.: Ultrasound features of a symptomatic splenic hemangioma. J Clin Ultrasound 12:95, 1984.

Martin JW: Congenital splenic cysts. Am J Surg 96:302, 1958.

Roshkow JE, Sanders LM: Acute splenic sequestration crisis in two adults with sickle cell disease: US, CT, and MR imaging findings. Radiology 177:723, 1990.

Schölmerich J, Volk BA: Differential diagnosis of anechoic/hypoechoic lesions in the abdomen detected by ultrasound. J Clin Ultrasound 14:339, 1986.

Sirinek KR, Evans WE: Nonparasitic splenic cysts. Am J Surg 126:8, 1973.

MASSES

Common

Hematoma
Abscess

Uncommon

Lymphoma
Melanoma metastasis
Ovarian metastasis
Colonic metastasis

CALCIFICATIONS

Common

TB
Histoplasmosis
Splenic artery atherosclerosis
Posttraumatic cyst

Uncommon

Hydatid cyst
Phleboliths
Hemangioma
Brucellosis
Sickle cell disease
Thorotrast
Infarct, healed
Healed abscess

Brauner M, Buffard MD, Jeantils V, et al.: Sonography and computed tomography of macroscopic tuberculosis of the liver. J Clin Ultrasound 17:563, 1989.

Stomach

WALL THICKENING

Common	Comment
Carcinoma	
Ulcer	
Gastritis	

Uncommon

Hematoma	
Leiomyosarcoma	
Lymphoma	
Metastases	
Leiomyoma	
Enteric duplication	Cystic
Giant folds	
Ménétrier's disease	Protein losing enteropathy; hypertrophic gastropathy
Heterotopic pancreas	Forms cystic lesions in wall
Adenoma	
Hypertrophic pyloric stenosis	
Schönlein-Henoch purpura	
Ischemia	
Crohn's disease	
Postradiation	
Zollinger-Ellison syndrome	
Lipoma	
Neurofibroma	

Claudon M, Verain AL, Bigard MA, et al.: Cyst formation in gastric heterotopic pancreas: Report of two cases. Radiology 169:659, 1988.

Gassner I, Strasser K, Bart G, et al.: Sonographic appearance of Ménétrier's disease in a child. J Ultrasound Med 9:537, 1990.

Joharjy IA, Mustafa MA, Zaidi AJ: Fluid-aided sonography of the stomach and duodenum in the diagnosis of peptic ulcer disease in adult patients. J Ultrasound Med 9:77, 1990.

Morimoto K, Hashimoto T, Choi S, et al.: Ultrasonographic evaluation of intramural gastric and duodenal hematoma in hemophiliacs. J Clin Ultrasound 16:108, 1988.

Parker LA, Vincent LM, Ryan FP, et al.: Primary lymphoma of the ascending colon: Sonographic demonstration. J Clin Ultrasound 14:221, 1986.

Tomooka Y, Onitsuka H, Goya T, et al.: Ultrasonography of benign gastric ulcers: Characteristic features and sequential follow-ups. J Ultrasound Med 8:513, 1989.

Weinberg B, Rao PS, Shah KD, et al.: Ultrasound demonstration of an intramural leiomyoma of the gastric cardia with pathologic correlation. J Clin Ultrasound 16:580, 1988.

Worlicek H, Dunz D, Engelhard K: Ultrasonic examination of the wall of the fluid-filled stomach. J Clin Ultrasound 17:5, 1989.

MASSES

Common

Gastric cancer

Uncommon

Glomus tumor
Bezoar
Leiomyoma
Leiomyosarcoma

Bidula MM, Rifkin MD, McCoy RL: Ultrasonography of gastric phytobezoar. J Clin Ultrasound 14:49, 1986.

Dupuy DE, Raptopoulos V, Meyer D, et al.: Sonographic findings in glomus tumor of the stomach. J Clin Ultrasound 17:219, 1989.

Bowel

WALL THICKENING

Common	Comment
Carcinoma	
Intussusception	
Lymphoma	
Hematoma	
Inflammatory disease	
Crohn's disease	Usually hypoechoic wall
Ulcerative colitis	Thick in active disease
Low albumin state	

Uncommon	
Leiomyosarcoma	
Typhlitis	Seen in leukemia, lymphoma
Schönlein-Henoch purpura	
Diverticulitis	
Whipple's disease	May give target lesions
Pseudomembranous colitis	Due to antibiotic use
Duodenal ulcer	Thickening of duodenum
Amebic colitis	Usually ascending colon
Campylobacter jejuni enteritis	May thicken terminal ileum
Adenoma	
Postradiation	
Ischemia	
Pancreatitis	May thicken adjacent bowel
Strongyloidiasis	
Lymphangioma	
Adjacent abscess	
Amyloidosis	
Giardia	
Behçet's syndrome	
Ameba	
Tuberculosis	
Metastases	
Carcinoid tumors	
Polyposis syndrome	

Albano O, Carrieri V, Vinciguerra V, et al.: Ultrasonic findings in Whipple's disease. J Clin Ultrasound 12:286, 1984.

Bolondi L, Ferrentino M, Trevisani F, et al: Sonographic appearance of pseudomembranous colitis. J Ultrasound Med 4:489, 1985.

Burke LF, Clark E: Ilio-colic intussusception: A case report. J Clin Ultrasound 5:346, 1977.

Chau WK, Na AT, Loh IW, et al.: Real-time ultrasound diagnosis of intramural intestinal hematoma. J Clin Ultrasound 17:382, 1989.

Glass-Royal MC, Choyke PL, Gootenberg JE, et al.: Sonography in the diagnosis of neutropenic colitis. J Ultrasound Med 6:671, 1987.

Joharjy IA, Mustafa MA, Zaidi AJ: Fluid-aided sonography of the stomach and duodenum in the diagnosis of peptic ulcer disease in adult patients. J. Ultrasound Med 9:77, 1990.

Lee TC, Brickman FE, Avecilla LS: Ultrasound diagnosis of intramural intestinal hematoma. J Clin Ultrasound 5:423, 1977.

Limberg B: Diagnosis of acute ulcerative colitis and colonic Crohn's disease by colonic sonography. J Clin Ultrasound 17:25, 1989.

Miller JH, Hindman BW, Lam AHK: Ultrasound in the evaluation of small bowel lymphoma in children. Radiology 135:409, 1980.

Miyamoto Y, Fukuda Y, Urushibara K, et al.: Ultrasonographic findings in duodenum caused by Schönlein-Henoch purpura. J Clin Ultrasound 17:299, 1989.

Morimoto K, Hashimoto T, Choi S, et al.: Ultrasonographic evaluation of intramural gastric and duodenal hematoma in hemophiliacs. J Clin Ultrasound 16:108, 1988.

Parienty RA, Lepreux JF, Gruson B: Sonographic and CT features of ileocolic intussusception. AJR 136:608, 1981.

Puylaert JBCM, Lalisang RI, van der Werf SDJ, et al.: *Campylobacter* ileocolitis mimicking acute appendicitis: Differentiation with graded-compression US. Radiology 166:737, 1988.

Skaane P, Skjennald A: Ultrasonic features of ileocecal intussusception. J Clin Ultrasound 17:590, 1989.

Sonnenberg A, Erckenbrecht J, Peter P, et al.: Detection of Crohn's disease by ultrasound. Gastroenterology 83:430, 1982.

Verbanck J, Lambrecht S, Rutgeerts L, et al.: Can sonography diagnose acute colonic diverticulitis in patients with acute intestinal inflammation? A prospective study. J Clin Ultrasound 17:661, 1989.

Worlicek H, Lutz H, Heyder N, et al.: Ultrasound findings in Crohn's disease and ulcerative colitis: A prospective study. J Clin Ultrasound 15:153, 1987.

MASSES

Common

Feces
Cancer

Uncommon

Polyp
Foreign body
Ascaris

Peck RJ: Ultrasonography of intestinal ascaris. J Clin Ultrasound 18:741, 1990.

Skaane P: Ultrasonic demonstration of a pedunculated colonic polyp. J Clin Ultrasound 15:204, 1987.

Pelvis

MASSES, MALE

Common	Comment
Hematoma	
Abscess	
Metastatic nodes	

Uncommon

Urinomas	
Lymphoceles	
Pelvic lipomatosis	Bilateral echogenic masses
Seminal vesicle abscess	
Mucocele of appendix	Complex mass with calcified rim
Angiomyxoma of cervix	Mostly cystic
Fibromyxoma	Homogeneous; solid; echogenic
Undescended testicle	
Pars infravaginalis gubernaculum	Termination of cord that extends from testis to scrotum; may see mass in undescended testis
Cystic mesothelioma	Benign; usually seen in women
Prostate cancer	

Athey PA, Hacken JB, Estrada R: Sonographic appearance of mucocele of the appendix. J Clin Ultrasound 12:333, 1984.

Lee SB, Lee F, Solomon MH, et al.: Seminal vesicle abscess: Diagnosis by transrectal ultrasound. J Clin Ultrasound 14:546, 1986.

O'Neil JD, Ros PR, Storm BL, et al.: Cystic mesothelioma of the peritoneum. Radiology 170:333, 1989.

Rosenfield AT, Blair DN, McCarthy S, et al.: The pars infravaginalis gubernaculi: Importance in the identification of the undescended testis. AJR 153:775, 1989.

Yaghoobian J, Zinn D, Ramanathan K, et al.: Ultrasound and computed tomographic findings in aggressive angiomyxoma of the uterine cervix. J Ultrasound Med 6:209, 1987.

Yoshino MT, Mar DY, Hunter TB: Sonographic demonstration of a pelvic fibromyxoma. J Ultrasound Med 4:365, 1985.

Bladder

MASSES

Common	Comment
Transitional cell carcinoma	
Blood clot	
Cystitis	May give focal wall thickening
Stones	May adhere to bladder wall

Uncommon

Ureterocele	Cystic
Foley catheter balloon	May dissect partially through bladder wall
Bladder diverticulum	
Pheochromocytoma	
Endometriosis	
Chloroma	Due to leukemia
Metastases	
Neurofibroma	
Extension of prostate cancer	
Foreign body	
Wall hematoma	
Polyp	
Fungus ball	
Leiomyoma	
Leiomyosarcoma	
Schistosomiasis	

Fornage BD, Rifkin MD, Lemaire AD, et al.: Bladder metastasis of gastric carcinoma: Diagnosis by sonography. J Clin Ultrasound 12:578, 1984.

Hightower DR, Laing FC, Jeffrey RB: A tandem guide for renal biopsy. J Ultrasound Med 4:441, 1985.

Kumar R, Haque AK, Cohen MS: Endometriosis of the urinary bladder: Demonstration by sonography. J Clin Ultrasound 12:363, 1984.

McLeod AJ, Lewis E, Cox D: Chloroma of the urinary bladder: Sonographic findings. J Clin Ultrasound 12:434, 1984.

Parisi L, Bigagli M, Nicita G, et al.: Detection of a pheochromocytoma of the urinary bladder by ultrasonography. J Clin Ultrasound 11:215, 1983.

Shapeero LG, Vordermark JS: Bladder neurofibromatosis in childhood: Noninvasive imaging. J Ultrasound Med 9:177, 1990.

WALL THICKENING

Common

Comment

Transitional cell carcinoma
Blood clot — Moves with position change
Cystitis
Neurogenic bladder

Uncommon

Secondary to diverticulitis of bowel
Cyclophosphamide induced cystitis
Crohn's disease involvement of — Look for adherent bowel
   bladder
Colovesical fistula
Vesicovaginal fistula
Cystitis glandularis — Associated with pelvic lipomatosis
Candida cystitis
Extension of prostate cancer
Bladder outlet obstruction
Malakoplakia
Leukoplakia
Neurofibroma
Hemangioma
Schistosomiasis
Pheochromocytoma
Endometriosis
Adjacent abscess
Hematoma in wall

Boag GS, Nolan RL: Sonographic features of urinary bladder involvement in regional enteritis. J Ultrasound Med 7:125, 1988.

Carrington BM, Johnson RJ: Vesicovaginal fistula: Ultrasound delineation and pathological correlation. J Clin Ultrasound 18:674, 1990.

Chen SS, Chou YH, Tiu CM, et al.: Sonographic features of colovesical fistula. J Clin Ultrasound 18:589, 1990.

Duffis AW, Weinberg B, Diakoumakis EE: A case of cystitis glandularis with associated pelvic lipomatosis: Ultrasound evaluation. J Clin Ultrasound 18:733, 1990.

Goodling GAW: Sonography of *Candida albicans* cystitis. J Ultrasound Med 8:121, 1989.

Suzuki T, Yasumoto M, Shibuya H, et al.: Sonography of cyclophosphamide hemorrhagic cystitis: A report of two cases. J Clin Ultrasound 16:183, 1988.

Uterus

ENLARGED

Common	Comment
Pregnancy	
Postpartum state	
Leiomyomas	

Uncommon

Carcinoma	
Hydrometrocolpos	Hourglass configuration with fluid in vagina and uterus
Arteriovenous malformation (AVM) of uterus	
Adenomyosis	Normal texture of myometrium and endometrium

Ali GM, Kordorff R, Franke D: Ultrasound volumetry in hematometrocolpos. J Clin Ultrasound 17:257, 1988.

Baltarowich OH, Kurtz AB, Pennell RG, et al.: Pitfalls in the sonographic diagnosis of uterine fibroids. AJR 151:725, 1988.

Diwan RV, Brennan JN, Selim MA, et al.: Sonographic diagnosis of arteriovenous malformation of the uterus and pelvis. J Clin Ultrasound 11:295, 1983.

Siedler D, Laing FC, Jeffrey RB, et al.: Uterine adenomyosis: A difficult sonographic diagnosis. J Ultrasound Med 6:345, 1987.

MASSES

Common	Comment
Leiomyomata	Variable sonographic appearance
Carcinoma	

Uncommon

Metastases to uterus	
Adenomyosis	May appear as irregular sonolucencies in endometrium
Myolipoma	Echogenic
Leiomyosarcoma	

Baltarowich OH, Kurtz AB, Pennell RG, et al.: Pitfalls in the sonographic diagnosis of uterine fibroids. AJR 151:725, 1988.

Lehrman BJ, Nisenbaum HL, Glasser SA, et al.: Uterine myolipoma: Magnetic resonance imaging, computed tomographic, and ultrasound appearance. J Ultrasound Med 9:665, 1990.

THICKENED ENDOMETRIUM

Common

Comment

Endometrial hyperplasia
Retained products of conception
Inflammatory disease
Endometrial carcinoma
Gestational trophoblastic disease
Hematometra
Pyometra

Uncommon

Cervical pregnancy
Adenomyosis   Sonolucencies in endometrium

Bader-Armstrong B, Shah Y, Rubens D: Use of ultrasound and magnetic resonance imaging in the diagnosis of cervical pregnancy. J Clin Ultrasound 17:283, 1989.

Fleischer AC, Kalemeris CG, Entman SS: Sonographic depiction of the endometrium during normal cycles. Ultrasound Med Biol 12:271, 1986.

Fleischer AC, Kalemeris CG, Machin JE, et al.: Sonographic depiction of normal and abnormal endometrium with histopathologic correlation. J Ultrasound Med 5:445, 1986.

Forrest TS, Elyaderans MK, Muilenberg RI, et al.: Cyclical endometrial changes: US assessment with histologic correlation. Radiology 167:233, 1988.

Lister JE, Kane GJ, Ehrmann RL, et al.: Ultrasound appearance of adenomyosis mimicking adenocarcinoma in a postmenopausal woman. J Clin Ultrasound 16:519, 1988.

Malpani A, Singer J, Wolverson MK, et al.: Endometrial hyperplasia: Value of endometrial thickness in ultrasonographic diagnosis and clinical significance. J Clin Ultrasound 18:173, 1990.

ENDOMETRIAL FLUID

Common   ## Comment

Endometritis
Retained products of conception
Incomplete abortion
Pelvic inflammatory disease (PID)
Cervical obstruction   Frequently a result of tumor

Uncommon

Endometrial carcinoma
Adenomyosis
After perforation
Imperforate hymen
Cervical carcinoma

Cunat JS, Dunne MG, Butler M: Sonographic diagnosis of uterine perforation following suction curettage. J Clin Ultrasound 12:108, 1984.
Lister JE, Kane GJ, Ehrmann RL, et al.: Ultrasound appearance of adenomyosis mimicking adenocarcinoma in a postmenopausal woman. J Clin Ultrasound 16:519, 1988.
Trigaux JP, Marchandise B, Schoevaerdts JC, et al.: Partial abnormal infradiaphragmatic pulmonary venous connection visualized by two-dimensional abdominal ultrasonography. J Clin Ultrasound 12:425, 1984.

ENDOMETRIAL SHADOWING

Common   ## Comment

Gas
Intrauterine device (IUD)
Calcified fibroids
Retained products of conception

Uncommon

Osteoid tissue   Prior pregnancies or inflammation

Baltarowich OH, Kurtz AB, Pennell RG, et al.: Pitfalls in the sonographic diagnosis of uterine fibroids. AJR 151:725, 1988.
Oi RH, McGahan JP, Kanwit ED: Ultrasonographic identification of osteoid tissue in utero. J Clin Ultrasound 11:385, 1983.

Ovaries and Adnexa

ENLARGED

Common

Normal

Ectopic pregnancy
Follicular cysts
PID
Corpus luteum cyst of pregnancy
Carcinoma
Follicle

Comment

Up to 12 cc in reproductive-age
women

Uncommon

Polycystic ovaries
Metastases to ovary
Teratoma
Theca lutein cysts   Bilateral
Ovarian torsion
Brenner tumor of ovary   May be calcified
Fibroma/thecoma of ovary
Dysgerminoma
Torsion of ovary   Usually has cysts
Fibrosarcoma
Leukemic infiltration
Pelvic kidney simulating ovary
Adnexal abscess adjacent to ovary
Endometrioma simulating ovary
McCune-Albright syndrome

Athey PA, Malone RS: Sonography of ovarian fibromas/thecomas. J Ultrasound Med 6:431, 1987.
Athey PA, Siegel MF: Sonographic features of Brenner tumor of the ovary. J Ultrasound Med 6:367, 1987.
Graif M, Itzchak Y: Sonographic evaluation of ovarian torsion in childhood and adolescence. AJR 150:647, 1988.
Helvie MA, Silver TM: Ovarian torsion: Sonographic evaluation. J Clin Ultrasound 17:327, 1989.
Sheth S, Fishman EK, Buck JL, et al.: The variable sonographic appearances of ovarian teratomas: Correlation with CT. AJR 151:331, 1988.

CYSTIC OR COMPLEX OVARY OR ADNEXAL MASS

Common

Follicle
Follicular cysts
Cystadenoma
Cystadenocarcinoma
Corpus luteum cyst of pregnancy
PID
Ectopic pregnancy
Pelvic lymphadenopathy

Uncommon

	Comment
Theca lutein cysts	
Mucocele of appendix	
Ovarian torsion	Enlarged ovary, usually with cysts
Fallopian tube carcinoma	
Duplication cyst of bowel	
Cystic mesothelioma	Benign
Ovarian varicocele	
Polycystic ovarian	Many with this disease have normal-sized ovaries
Pelvic varices	
AVM of uterus and pelvis	
Peritoneal inclusion cyst	
Ovarian vein thrombophlebitis	Usually puerperal
Angiomyoma of cervix	Mostly cystic
Brenner tumor of ovary	May be calcified
Hemorrhagic cyst	
Endometrioma	
Leukemic infiltration	
Hydrosalpinx	
Teratoma	May be hypoechoic, hyperechoic, or mixed
Degenerated leiomyoma	
Anterior meningocele	
Pelvic kidney	

Ajjimakorn S, Bhamarapravati Y, Israngura N: Ultrasound appearance of fallopian tube carcinoma. J Clin Ultrasound 16:516, 1988.

Athey PA, Diment DD: The spectrum of sonographic findings in endometriomas. J Ultrasound Med 8:487, 1989.

Athey PA, Siegel MF: Sonographic features of Brenner tumor of the ovary. J Ultrasound Med 6:367, 1987.

Bahia JO, Wilson MH: Mucocele of the appendix presenting as an adnexal mass. J Clin Ultrasound 17:62, 1989.

Cancelmo RP: Sonographic demonstration of multilocular peritoneal inclusion cyst. J Clin Ultrasound 11:334, 1983.

Caspi B, Schachter M, Lancet M: Infected duplication cyst of ileum masquerading as an adnexal abscess—ultrasonographic features. J Clin Ultrasound 17:431, 1989.

Diwan RV, Brennan JN, Selim MA, et al.: Sonographic diagnosis of arteriovenous malformation of the uterus and pelvis. J Clin Ultrasound 11:295, 1983.

Giacchetto C, Cotroneo GB, Marincolo F, et al.: Ovarian varicocele: Ultrasonic and phlebographic evaluation. J Clin Ultrasound 18:551, 1990.

Graif M, Itzchak Y: Sonographic evaluation of ovarian torsion in childhood and adolescence. AJR 150:647, 1988.

Helvie MA, Silver TM: Ovarian torsion: Sonographic evaluation. J Clin Ultrasound 17:327, 1989.

Hoffer FA, Kozakewich H, Colodny A, et al. Peritoneal inclusion cysts: Ovarian fluid in peritoneal adhesions. Radiology 169:189, 1988.

Nicolini U, Ferrazzi E, Bellotti M, et al.: The contribution of sonographic evaluation of ovarian size in patients with polycystic ovarian disease. J Ultrasound Med 4:347, 1985.

O'Neil JD, Ros PR, Storm BL, et al.: Cystic mesothelioma of the peritoneum. Radiology 170:333, 1989.

Reuter K, Cohen S, Daly D: Ultrasonic presentation of giant hydrosalpinges in asymptomatic patients. J Clin Ultrasound 15:45, 1987.

Sheth S, Fishman EK, Buck JL, et al.: The variable sonographic appearances of ovarian teratomas: Correlation with CT. AJR 151:331, 1988.

Warhit JM, Fagelman D, Goldman MA, et al.: Ovarian vein thrombophlebitis: Diagnosis by ultrasound and CT. J Clin Ultrasound 12:301, 1984.

Willard DA: Pelvic varices: Sonographic and surgical recognition. J Clin Ultrasound 16:265, 1988.

Yaghoobian J, Zinn D, Ramanathan K, et al.: Ultrasound and computed tomographic findings in aggressive angiomyxoma of the uterine cervix. J Ultrasound Med 6:209, 1987.

Yeh HC, Young TH, Greenberg ML: Leukemic pelvic lymphadenopathy simulating cystic ovarian lesion on sonogram. J Clin Ultrasound 12:177, 1984.

PELVIC MASSES DURING PREGNANCY

Common	Comment
Corpus luteum cyst	May appear complex or solid after hemorrhage
Cystadenoma of ovary	
Endometrioma	
Ectopic pregnancy	May occur simultaneously with intrauterine pregnancy (IUP)

Uncommon	
Cystadenocarcinoma of ovary	
Enteric cyst	
Theca lutein cysts	Bilateral
Leiomyoma, pedunculated	May appear extrauterine
Lymphoma	
Teratoma	
Hydrosalpinx	
Mesenteric cyst	
Ovarian carcinoma	
Pelvic kidney	
Urachal cysts	
Paraovarian cysts	
Appendiceal abscess	
Crohn's disease abscesses	
Echinococcal cysts	
Lymphocele	
Schwannoma	
Bowel loop	
Spleen	May prolapse into pelvis
Ovarian pregnancy	
Tubo-ovarian abscess	
Peritoneal cyst	
Inclusion cyst	

Athey PA, Jayson HT, Estrada R, et al.: Sonographic findings in primary ovarian pregnancy. J Clin Ultrasound 18:730, 1990.

Fleischer AC, Boehm FH, James AE, Jr.: Sonography and radiology of pelvic masses and other maternal disorders. Semin Roentgenol 17:172, 1982.

Rahatzad MT, Adamson D: A pictorial essay of pelvic and abdominal masses seen during pregnancy. J Clin Ultrasound 14:255, 1986.

ADNEXAL CALCIFICATIONS

Common

Dermoid
Prior abscess

Uncommon

Brenner tumor
Uterine leiomyoma
Calcified hematoma
Fibroma/thecoma of ovary

Athey PA, Malone RS: Sonography of ovarian fibromas/thecomas. J Ultrasound Med 6:431, 1987.
Athey PA, Siegel MF: Sonographic features of Brenner tumor of the ovary. J Ultrasound Med 6:367, 1987.
Sheth S, Fishman EK, Buck JL, et al.: The variable sonographic appearances of ovarian teratomas: Correlation with CT. AJR 151:331, 1988.

SOLID ADNEXAL MASS

Common

Enlarged normal ovary
Ectopic pregnancy
PID
Endometrioma

Uncommon

Hemorrhage into ovarian cyst
Ovarian carcinoma
Torsion of ovary
Leukemic infiltration of ovary
Fallopian tube carcinoma
Metastatic disease
Rectal mass protruding to adnexa
Blood in cul-de-sac
Drop-metastasis in cul-de-sac
Appendiceal abscess
Teratoma

Athey PA, Diment DD: The spectrum of sonographic findings in endometriomas. J Ultrasound Med 8:487, 1989.

Baltarowich OH, Kurtz AB, Pasto ME, et al.: The spectrum of sonographic findings in hemorrhagic ovarian cysts. AJR 148:901, 1987.

Meyer JS, Kim CS, Price HM, et al.: Ultrasound presentation of primary carcinoma of the fallopian tube. J Clin Ultrasound 15:132, 1987.

Sheth S, Fishman EK, Buck JL, et al.: The variable sonographic appearances of ovarian teratomas: Correlation with CT. AJR 151:331, 1988.

Adrenal Glands

MASSES

Common	Comment
Hyperplasia	Usually bilateral
Adenomas	Usually unilateral
Metastases	Solid or complex

Uncommon	
Cysts	May be calcified
Abscesses	
Ganglioneuromas	
Pheochromocytomas	May see capsule; 10% bilateral
Adrenal cortical carcinoma	
Invasion from renal tumor	
Prominent diaphragmatic crus	
Myelolipoma	Complex mass with echogenic components
Neuroblastoma	
Lymphoma	
Hemorrhage	
Hydatid disease	

Miller EI, Dickerson RW: Sonographic appearance of myelolipoma: Demonstration of adrenal and pelvic lesions. J Clin Ultrasound 11:179, 1983.

Musante F, Derchi LE, Zappasodi F, et al.: Myelolipoma of the adrenal gland: Sonographic and CT features. AJR 151:961, 1988.

Vicks BS, Perusek M, Johnson J, et al.: Primary adrenal lymphoma: CT and sonographic appearances. J Clin Ultrasound 15:135, 1987.

CYSTS

	Comment
Parasitic	Usually hydatid
Epithelial	Cystic adenomas most common
Endothelial	Most common adrenal cyst
Pseudocysts	Occur after hemorrhage
Pyogenic cyst	
Lymphoma	

Barki Y, Eilig I, Moses M, et al.: Sonographic diagnosis of a large hemorrhagic adrenal cyst in an adult. J Clin Ultrasound 15:194, 1987.

Okafo BA, Nickel C, Morales A: Pyogenic cyst of adrenal gland. Urology 21:619, 1983.

Vicks BS, Perusek M, Johnson J, et al.: Primary adrenal lymphoma: CT and sonographic appearances. J Clin Ultrasound 15:135, 1987.

CALCIFICATIONS

Common	Comment
Posthemorrhage	
TB	

Uncommon	
Neuroblastoma	
Ganglioneuroma	
Wolman's disease	Inherited
Carcinoma	
Histoplasmosis	
Pheochromocytoma	Rarely calcified

Kidney

ENLARGED BILATERALLY, SMOOTH CONTOUR

Common

Hydronephrosis
Glomerulonephritis
Acute tubular necrosis
Response to diuretics and contrast
   materials

Uncommon

Preeclampsia
IgA glomerulosclerosis
Glomerulosclerosis of heroin abuse
Membranous glomerulonephritis
Polyarteritis nodosa
Lupus erythematosus
Wegener's granulomatosis
Allergic angiitis
Diabetic glomerulosclerosis
Goodpasture's syndrome
Schönlein-Henoch purpura
Thrombotic thrombocytopenic purpura
Glomerulonephritis of subacute
   bacterial endocarditis (SBE)
Amyloidosis
Multiple myeloma
Acute cortical necrosis
Leukemic infiltration
Acute interstitial nephritis
Acute urate nephropathy
Homozygous-S disease
Hemophilia
With cirrhosis
With acromegaly
Fabry's disease
Bilateral duplicated system
Beckwith-Wiedemann syndrome

Comment

Echogenic

Davidson AJ: *Radiology of the Kidney*. Philadelphia, WB Saunders, 1985.
Schutz K, Siffring PA, Forrest TS, et al.: Serial renal sonographic changes in preeclampsia. J Ultrasound Med 9:415, 1990.

ENLARGED UNILATERALLY, SMOOTH CONTOUR

Common

Renal vein thrombosis
Obstruction
Acute pyelonephritis
Compensatory hypertrophy
Duplicated system

Uncommon

Acute arterial infarct

Davidson AJ: *Radiology of the Kidney.* Philadelphia, WB Saunders, 1985.

ENLARGED UNILATERALLY, MULTIFOCAL LESIONS

Common

Multiple cysts

Comment

Uncommon

Xanthogranulomatous pyelonephritis	Usually has stone
Malakoplakia	Multiple, hypoechoic masses
Multicystic dysplastic kidney	Disorganized with anechoic masses
TB	
Metastases	
Multiple, primary tumors	

Davidson AJ: *Radiology of the Kidney.* Philadelphia, WB Saunders, 1985.

ENLARGED BILATERALLY, MULTIFOCAL LESIONS

Common	Comment
APKD	
Multiple, simple cysts	

Uncommon	
Acquired cystic disease	Dialysis patients
Hodgkin's disease/lymphoma of kidney	
Bilateral tumors	
Multiple hamartomas	As in tuberous sclerosis

Davidson AJ: *Radiology of the Kidney.* Philadelphia, WB Saunders, 1985.

SMALL, UNILATERAL, SMOOTH CONTOUR

Common	Comment
Reflux atrophy	Often has irregular contour

Uncommon	
Renal artery stenosis or ischemia	
Chronic renal infarction	
Radiation nephritis	
Congenital hypoplasia	
Postobstructive atrophy	
Postinflammatory atrophy	
Heminephrectomy	

Davidson AJ: *Radiology of the Kidney.* Philadelphia, WB Saunders, 1985.

SMALL, BILATERAL, SMOOTH CONTOUR

Common	*Comment*
Hypertensive nephropathy	
Generalized arteriosclerosis	
Nephrosclerosis	

Uncommon

Atheroembolic renal disease	
Chronic glomerulonephritis	
Renal papillary necrosis	
Alport's syndrome	
Medullary cystic disease	
Late amyloidosis	
Hypotension	
Bilateral renal artery stenosis	
Radiation nephritis	
Postobstructive atrophy, bilateral	
Postinflammatory atrophy	Usually not smooth
Reflux atrophy	Usually not smooth
Bilateral infarcts	Usually not smooth
Renal cortical necrosis	
Lead poisoning	

Davidson AJ: *Radiology of the Kidney.* Philadelphia, WB Saunders, 1985.

CYSTIC MASSES

Common	*Comment*
Simple cysts	
Focal hydronephrosis	
Abscesses	
Hematomas	
Peripelvic cysts	

Uncommon

Adenocarcinoma	
Urinoma	
Vascular malformations	
Focal pyelonephritis	
Xanthogranulomata	
Renal artery aneurysm	
Calyceal diverticula	
Cyst with mural tumor	
Renal pyramids	Rarely meet cystic criteria
APKD	
Multicystic dysplastic kidney	
Postdialysis cysts	
Angiomyolipoma	Rarely anechoic
Urinoma	Not intrarenal
Renal artery pseudoaneurysm	After biopsy
Lymphangioma	Multilocular cystic
Metastases	

Behan M, Martin EC, Muecke EC, et al.: Myelolipoma of the adrenal: Two cases with ultrasound and CT findings. Am J Roentgenol 129:993, 1977.

Hantmann SS, Barie JJ, Glendening TB, et al.: Giant renal artery aneurysm mimicking a simple cyst on ultrasound. J Clin Ultrasound 10:136, 1982.

Hartmann DS, Goldman SM, Friedman AC, et al.: Angiomyolipoma: Ultrasonic-pathologic correlation. Radiology 139:451, 1981.

Jacobs JE, Sussman SK, Glickstein MF: Renal lymphangiomyoma—A rare cause of a multiloculated renal mass. AJR 152:307, 1988.

Lee TG, Henderson SC, Freeny PC, et al.: Ultrasound findings of renal angiomyolipoma. J Clin Ultrasound 6:150, 1978.

Schölmerich J, Volk BA: Differential diagnosis of anechoic/hypoechoic lesions in the abdomen detected by ultrasound. J Clin Ultrasound 14:339, 1986.

Suramo I, Päivänsalo M, Leinonen A, et al.: The sonographic images of hypernephromas. Fortschr Roentgenstr 135:649, 1981.

Weissman J, Giyanani VL, Landreneau MD, et al.: Postbiopsy arterial pseudoaneurysm in a renal allograft: Detection by duplex sonography. J Ultrasound Med 7:515, 1988.

COMPLEX MASSES

Common	Comment
Adenocarcinoma	
Hematomas	
Abscesses	

Uncommon

Infarcts	Especially when hemorrhagic
Infected cysts	
Hemorrhagic cysts	
Pyonephrosis	
Peripelvic cysts	
Xanthogranulomatous pyelonephritis	Variable echogenicity
Focal bacterial pyelonephritis	May be hyperechoic
Angiomyolipoma	Variable appearance
Lymphoma	
Transitional cell carcinoma	
Multicystic dysplastic kidney	
Lymphangioma	Multilocular cystic

Jacobs JE, Sussman SK, Glickstein MF: Renal lymphangiomyoma—A rare cause of a multiloculated renal mass. AJR 152:307, 1988.

SOLID MASSES

Common	*Comment*
Adenocarcinoma	Usually hypoechoic

Uncommon

Lymphoma	
Hematoma	
Calcified cyst	
Abscess	
Angiomyolipoma	Frequently echogenic
Transitional cell carcinoma	
Sinus lipomatosis	
Leukemic infiltrate	
Neurofibroma	
Extramedullary hematopoiesis	
Carcinoid of kidney	Echogenic

McKeown DK, Nguyen G-K, Rudrick B, et al.: Carcinoid of the kidney: Radiologic findings. AJR 150:143, 1988.

Shawker TH, Hill M, Hill S, et al.: Ultrasound appearance of extramedullary hematopoiesis. J Ultrasound Med 6:283, 1987.

RENAL PELVIC MASSES

Common	Comment
Transitional cell carcinoma	
Stones	
Peripelvic cyst	

Uncommon

Neurofibroma
Squamous cell carcinoma of pelvis
Adenocarcinoma of pelvis
Lymphoma
Renal vein varices
Fungus balls
Hematoma
Matrix calculus   May not shadow

Bick RJ, Bryan PJ: Sonographic demonstration of thickened renal pelvic mucosa/submucosa in mixed candida infection. J Clin Ultrasound 15:333, 1987.

Kauzlaric D, Barmeir E: Ultrasonic detection of renal pelvic and ureteric varices. J Clin Ultrasound 12:569, 1984.

LeCheong L, Khan AN, Bisset RAL: Sonographic features of a renal pelvic neurofibroma. J Clin Ultrasound 18:129, 1990.

Maklad NF, Chuang VP, Doust BD, et al.: Ultrasonic characterization of solid renal lesions: Echographic, angiographic, and pathologic correlation. Radiology 123:733, 1977.

Mullholland SG, Arger PH, Goldberg BB, et al.: Ultrasonic differentiation of renal pelvic filling defects. J Urol 122:14, 1979.

Ruchman RB, Yeh HC, Mitty HA, et al.: Ultrasonographic and computed tomographic features of renal sinus lymphoma. J Clin Ultrasound 16:35, 1988.

Schmitt GH, Hsu AS: Renal fungus balls: Diagnosis by ultrasound and percutaneous antegrade pyelography and brush biopsy in a premature infant. J Ultrasound Med 4:155, 1985.

Subramanyan BR, Raghavendra BN, Madamba MR: Renal transitional cell carcinoma: Sonographic and pathologic correlation. J Clin Ultrasound 10:203, 1982.

Zwirewich CV, Buckley AR, Kidney MR, et al.: Renal matrix calculus: Sonographic appearance. J Ultrasound Med 9:61, 1990.

ABNORMAL ECHOGENICITY

Increased Cortical Echogenicity Compared to Medulla

Common

Acute glomerulonephritis
Chronic glomerulonephritis
Nephrosclerosis
Diabetic nephropathy
Acute tubular necrosis
Transplant rejection

Uncommon

Lupus erythematosus
Alport's syndrome
Papillary necrosis
Preeclampsia
Amyloidosis
Nephrocalcinosis
Renal vein thrombosis
AIDS
Acute cortical necrosis
Leukemic infiltration
Beckwith-Wiedemann syndrome

Comment

Calcified, echogenic cortex
Bilateral

Hamper UM, Goldblum LE, Hutchins GM, et al.: Renal involvement in AIDS: Sonographic-pathologic correlation. AJR 150:1321, 1988.

Kumari-Subaiya S, Lee WJ, Festa R, et al.: Sonographic findings in leukemic renal disease. J Clin Ultrasound 12:465, 1984.

LeQuesne GW: Ultrasonic detection of glomerular disease. AJR 130:96, 1978.

Rochester D, Aronson AJ, Bowie JD, et al.: Ultrasonic appearance of acute poststreptococcal glomerulonephritis. J Clin Ultrasound 6:49, 1978.

Rosenberg ER, Trought WS, Kirks DR, et al.: Ultrasonic diagnosis of renal vein thrombosis in neonates. AJR 134:35, 1980.

Schutz K, Siffring PA, Forrest TS, et al.: Serial renal sonographic changes in preeclampsia. J Ultrasound Med 9:415, 1990.

Shapeero LG, Vordermark JS: Papillary necrosis causing hydronephrosis in the renal allograft: Sonographic findings. J Ultrasound Med 8:579, 1989.

Shuman WP, Mack LA, Rogers JV: Diffuse nephrocalcinosis: Hyperechoic sonographic appearance. AJR 136:830, 1981.

Sty JR, Starshak RJ, Hubbard AM: Acute renal cortical necrosis in hemolytic uremic syndrome. J Clin Ultrasound 11:175, 1983.

Subramanyam BR: Renal amyloidosis in juvenile rheumatoid arthritis sonographic features. AJR 136:411, 1981.

Increased Echogenicity, No Distinction Between Cortex and Medulla

Common	Comment

Common

Chronic pyelonephritis
Chronic glomerulonephritis

Uncommon

Focal acute bacterial nephritis
AIDS   Usually in drug users
Healing infarct
Infantile polycystic kidney disease
  (IPKD)
Renal tubular ectasia
APKD
Medullary cystic disease

Boal DK, Teele RL: Sonography of infantile polycystic kidney disease. AJR 135:575, 1980.

Hamper UM, Goldblum LE, Hutchins GM, et al.: Renal involvement in AIDS: Sonographic-pathologic correlation. AJR 150:1321, 1988.

Kay CJ, Rosenfield AT, Taylor KJW, et al.: Ultrasonic characteristics of chronic atrophic pyelonephritis. AJR 132:47, 1979.

Lee JKT, McClennan BL, Melson GL, et al.: Acute focal bacterial nephritis: Emphasis on gray scale sonography and computed tomography. AJR 135:87, 1980.

Rosenfield AT, Glickman MG, Taylor KJW, et al.: Acute focal bacterial nephritis (acute lobar nephroma). Radiology 132:553, 1979.

Yee JM, Raghavendra N, Horii SC, et al.: Abdominal sonography in AIDS: A review. J Ultrasound Med 8:705, 1989.

ECHOGENIC MEDULLA

Tamm-Horsefall proteinuria
Sepsis
Dehydration
Candida
Renal tubular necrosis
Williams syndrome
Gout
Sjögren's syndrome
Medullary sponge kidney
Primary aldosteronism
Lesch-Nyhan syndrome
Glycogen storage disease type I
Wilson's disease
Pseudo-Bartter's syndrome
Hypokalemia
Medullary nephrocalcinosis
   Hyperparathyroidism
   Chronic pyelonephritis
   Chronic glomerulonephritis
   Distal renal tubular acidosis
   Milk-alkali syndrome
   Malignancy with bone involvement
   Hypervitaminosis D
   Primary hypercalcemia
   Sarcoidosis
   Renal tubular acidosis

Cote G, Jequiers S, Kaplan P: Increased renal medullary echogenicity in patients with Williams syndrome. Pediatr Radiol 19:481, 1989.
Cramer BC, Jequiers S, de Chadarevian JP: Factors associated with renal parenchymal echogenicity in the newborn. J Ultrasound Med 5:633, 1986.

DECREASED CORTICAL ECHOGENICITY

	Comment
Acute pyelonephritis	One or more hypoechoic areas
Renal vein thrombosis	
Transplant rejection	
Lupus nephritis	Multiple cortical hypoechoic areas
Multicentric renal cell carcinoma	Multiple hypoechoic areas
Lymphoma of kidneys	Multiple hypoechoic areas

Longmaid HE, Rider E, Tymkiw J: Lupus nephritis: New sonographic findings. J Ultrasound Med 6:75, 1987.

INTERNAL ECHOGENIC AREAS

Common	Comment
Renal stones	
Renal calcifications	
Calcifications too small to shadow	

Uncommon

Renal gas	As seen in emphysematous pyelonephritis
Fat-filled postoperative cortical defect	Retroperitoneal fat fills in postoperative cortical defects
TB with calcifications	
Renal tubular acidosis	Medullary calcifications
Medullary sponge kidney	May not see calcifications
Hyperoxaluria	May give calcifications
Sarcoidosis	May give calcifications
Milk-alkali syndrome	Stones or calcifications
Hypervitaminosis D	Stones or calcifications
Hyperparathyroidism	Stones or calcifications
Calcification in cysts	
Calcification in adenocarcinoma	
Carcinoma with paraneoplastic syndrome	Especially lung or breast
Metastatic carcinoma to bone	May give calcifications
Calcification in xanthogranulomatous pyelonephritis	
Papillary necrosis	Sloughed papillae may calcify
Echinococcus with calcification	
Calcified multicystic dysplastic kidney	

Balsara VJ, Raval B, Maklad NF: Emphysematous pyelonephritis in a renal transplant: Sonographic and computed tomographic features. J Ultrasound Med 4:97, 1985.

Chou YH, Tiu CM, Chen TW, et al.: Emphysematous pyelonephritis in a polycystic kidney: Demonstration by ultrasound and computed tomography. J Ultrasound Med 9:355, 1990.

Papanicolaou N, Harbury OL, Pfister RC: Fat-filled postoperative renal cortical defects: Sonographic and CT appearance. AJR 151:503, 1988.

DILATED COLLECTING SYSTEM

Common

Urinary obstruction
Reflux

Uncommon

Infection causing aperistalsis
Diuresis
Distended bladder
Extrarenal pelvis
After relief of obstruction
After diuretics
After contrast injection
Overhydration
Megacalyces
Papillary necrosis
Diabetes insipidus
Postinflammatory calyceal clubbing
After ESWL

Kaude JV, Williams JL, Wright PG, et al.: Sonographic evaluation of the kidney following extracorporeal shock wave lithotripsy. J Ultrasound Med 6:299, 1987.
Shapeero LG, Vordermark JS: Papillary necrosis causing hydronephrosis in the renal allograft: Sonographic findings. J Ultrasound Med 8:579, 1989.

CONFUSED WITH DILATED COLLECTING SYSTEM

Common	*Comment*
Central renal cysts	
Parapelvic cysts	
Multiple simple cysts	

Uncommon

Lucent renal pyramids	
Lumbar meningomyelocele	
Pancreatic pseudocyst	
Renal artery aneurysm	
Sinus lipomatosis	Sinus fat may have variable echogenicity
Hypoechoic renal lymphoma	

WALL THICKENING OF COLLECTING SYSTEM

Rejection in transplants
Acute tubular necrosis
Urinary tract infection complicating
  hydronephrosis
Congenital hydronephrosis after
  pyeloplasty
Congenital hydronephrosis due to
  reflux
Total parenteral nutrition
Previously obstructed system
Chronic obstruction

Babcock DS: Sonography of wall thickening of the renal collecting system: A nonspecific finding. J Ultrasound Med 6:29, 1987.
Nicolet V, Carignan L, Dubuc G, et al.: Thickening of the renal collecting system: A nonspecific finding at US. Radiology 168:411, 1988.

ECHOES WITHIN COLLECTING SYSTEM

Common	Comment
Stones	
Blood clots	
Transitional cell carcinoma	
Infected obstructed system (pyonephrosis)	
Emphysematous pyelonephritis	Gas may produce echoes
Nephrostomy tube	
Stent	

Uncommon

Gas (emphysematous pyelonephritis)
Sloughed papillae

Chou YH, Tiu CM, Chen TW, et al.: Emphysematous pyelonephritis in a polycystic kidney: Demonstration by ultrasound and computed tomography. J Ultrasound Med 9:355, 1990.

ENLARGED RENAL VESSELS

Common	Comment
Renal AVM	Artery and vein both enlarged
Renal artery aneurysm	
Renal cell carcinoma	Especially if vessel is filled with tumor clot

PERIRENAL FLUID

Common

Blood, after trauma
Blood, after biopsy
Spontaneously decompressed
 obstructed system

Uncommon

Urinoma
Lymphocele
Perinephric abscess
Herniated bowel
Pancreatic pseudocysts
After percutaneous stone removal
Abscess
Blood associated with tumor or
 vascular abnormality

Belville JS, Morgentaler A, Loughlin KR, et al.: Spontaneous perinephric and subcapsular renal hemorrhage: Evaluation with CT, US, and angiography. Radiology 172:733, 1989.
Burks DD, Fleischer AC, Richie RE: Sonographic diagnosis of a perirenal transplant bowel hernia. J Ultrasound Med 4:677, 1985.

Kidney Transplant

ENLARGED

Acute tubular necrosis
Rejection
Hydronephrosis
Infection

Babcock DS, Slovis TL, Han BK, et al.: Renal transplants in children: Long-term follow-up using sonography. Radiology 156:165, 1985.
Frick MP, Feinberg SB, Sibley RK, et al.: Ultrasound in acute renal transplant rejection. Radiology 138:657, 1981.
Maklad NF: Ultrasonic evaluation of renal transplants. Semin Ultrasound 2:88, 1981.
Slovis TL, Babcock DS, Hricak H, et al.: Renal transplant rejection: Sonographic evaluation in children. Radiology 153:659, 1984.

INCREASED ECHOGENICITY

Obstruction
Rejection
Renal vein thrombosis

Babcock DS, Slovis TL, Han BK, et al.: Renal transplants in children: Long-term follow-up using sonography. Radiology 156:165, 1985.
Frick MP, Feinberg SB, Sibley RK, et al.: Ultrasound in acute renal transplant rejection. Radiology 138:657, 1981.
Maklad NF: Ultrasonic evaluation of renal transplants. Semin Ultrasound 2:88, 1981.
Slovis TL, Babcock DS, Hricak H, et al.: Renal transplant rejection: Sonographic evaluation in children. Radiology 153:659, 1984.

PERINEPHRIC FLUID

Normal within first 10 days
Abscess
Lymphocele
Hematoma
Urinoma
Ovarian cystadenoma
Herniated bowel

Burks DD, Fleischer AC, Richie RE: Sonographic diagnosis of a perirenal transplant bowel hernia. J Ultrasound Med 4:677, 1985.
Kliewer MA, Woodruff WW, Bowie JD: Mucinous cystadenoma simulating renal transplant lymphocele. J Clin Ultrasound 17:119, 1989.
Silver TM, Campbell D, Wicks JD, et al.: Peritransplant fluid collections: Ultrasound evaluation and clinical significance. Radiology 138:145, 1981.

MASSES

Lymphoma
Hematoma
Abscess
Herniated bowel

Burks DD, Fleischer AC, Richie RE: Sonographic diagnosis of a perirenal transplant bowel hernia. J Ultrasound Med 4:677, 1985.
Olcott EW, Goldstein RB, Salvatierra O: Lymphoma presenting as allograft hematoma in a renal transplant recipient. J Ultrasound Med 9:239, 1990.

Retroperitoneum

MASSES

Common	Comment
Lymphoma	
Hemorrhage	
Metastases	Frequently testicular carcinoma or lymphoma
Abscesses, especially psoas	

Uncommon

	Comment
Retroperitoneal fibrosis	Hypoechoic to anechoic; little retroaortic extension
Liposarcomas	Often echogenic
Lymphocele	
Cysts	
Leiomyosarcoma	
Hemangiopericytoma	
Teratomas	
Mucocele of appendix	Right lower quadrant (RLQ) mass; complex; rim calcification

---

Athey PA, Hacken JB, Estrada R: Sonographic appearance of mucocele of the appendix. J Clin Ultrasound 12:333, 1984.

CYSTIC LESIONS

Common	*Comment*
Aneurysms	
Abscesses	
Hematomas	
Metastases	

Uncommon

Urinomas	
Lymphoceles	
Varices	
Urachal cysts	
Sacral meningocele	
Retroperitoneal fibrosis	
Tumors, especially sarcomas	
Cystic lymphangioma	
Mucocele of appendix	Complex mass with calcified rim

Athey PA, Hacken JB, Estrada R: Sonographic appearance of mucocele of the appendix. J Clin Ultrasound 12:333, 1984.

Davidson AJ, Hartman DS: Lymphangioma of the retroperitoneum: CT and sonographic characteristics. Radiology 175:507, 1990.

Gould HR, Benjamin S, Alter AJ, et al.: Retroperitoneal varices simulating masses. Gastrointest Radiol 7:335, 1982.

McCreath GT, Macpherson P: Sonography in the diagnosis and management of anterior sacral meningocele. J Clin Ultrasound 8:133, 1980.

Radin R, Weiner S, Koenigsberg M, et al.: Retroperitoneal cystic lymphangioma. Am J Roentgenol 140:733, 1983.

Rossi L, Mandrioli R, Rossi A, et al.: Retroperitoneal cystic lymphangioma. Br J Radiol 55:676, 1982.

Schölmerich J, Volk BA: Differential diagnosis of anechoic/hypoechoic lesions in the abdomen detected by ultrasound. J Clin Ultrasound 14:339, 1986.

Williams BD, Fisk JD: Sonographic diagnosis of giant urachal cysts in the adult. Am J Roentgenol 136:417, 1981.

Scrotum

FLUID AND MASSES, EXTRATESTICULAR

Common

Comment

Primary hydrocele — Between two layers of tunica vaginalis

Reactive hydrocele — Due to tumor, trauma, infarction, inflammation

Varicoceles — Dilation of draining veins of pampiniform plexus

Ascites

Hematoceles

Spermatocele — Dilation of epididymal ducts

Epididymitis

Uncommon

Cysts

Herniated bowel

Epididymal cysts — Anywhere along course of epididymis

Pyoceles

Adenomatoid tumor — Usually from globus minor of epididymis; hyperechogenic or hypoechogenic

Extratesticular seminoma

Leiomyomas

Fibromas

Adrenal rests

Lipomas

Chronic epididymitis — Epididymal enlargement

Metastases

Rhabdomyosarcoma of funiculus

Sarcoidosis

Sperm granuloma

Mesothelioma of tunica vaginalis — Solid mass

Bowel herniation into scrotum — May have peristalsis

Polyorchidism

Fibrolipoma of cord

Lymphangioma

Mesothelioma of tunica albuginea

Aquino NM, Vazquez R, Matari H: Ultrasound demonstration of a benign mesothelioma of tunica vaginalis testis. J Clin Ultrasound 14:310, 1986.

Arger PH, Mulhern CB, Coleman BG, et al.: Prospective analysis of the value of scrotal ultrasound. Radiology 141:763, 1981.

Carroll BA, Gross DM: High frequency scrotal sonography. AJR 140:511, 1983.

Forsberg L, Olsson AM: Examination of the pathological scrotum with dynamic and static ultrasound. Br J Radiol 56:921, 1983.

Forte MD, Brant WE: Ultrasonographic detection of epididymal sarcoidosis. J Clin Ultrasound 16:191, 1988.

Goldberg RM, Chilcote W, Kay R, et al.: Sonographic findings in polyorchidism. J Clin Ultrasound 15:412, 1987.

Hricak H, Filly RA: Sonography of the scrotum. Invest Radiol 18:112, 1983.

Huben RP, Scarff JE, Schellhammer PE: Massive intrascrotal fibrolipoma. J Urol 129:154, 1983.

Kutchera WA, Bluth EI, Guice SL: Sonographic findings of a spermatic cord lipoma: Case report and review of the literature. J Ultrasound Med 6:457, 1987.

Martin B, Conte J: Ultrasonography of the acute scrotum. J Clin Ultrasound 15:37, 1987.

Orr DP, Skolnick ML: Sonographic examination of the abnormal scrotum. Clin Radiol 31:109, 1980.

Ramanathan K, Yaghoobian J, Pinck RL: Sperm granuloma. J Clin Ultrasound 14:155, 1986.

Solivetti FM, D'Ascenzo R, Molisso A, et al.: Rhabdomyosarcoma of the funiculus. J Clin Ultrasound 17:521, 1989.

Vick CW, Bird KI, Rosenfield AT, et al.: Scrotal masses with a uniformly hyperechoic pattern. Radiology 148:209, 1983.

CYSTIC MASS, EXTRATESTICULAR

Common   ## Comment

Hematoceles
Spermatoceles

Uncommon

Epididymal cysts	
Pyoceles	
Torsion of Giraldés' organ	Also known as paradidymis
Lymphocele	Seen usually after transplant
Herniation of bowel into scrotum	Look for peristalsis

Avner E, Ellis D, Jaffe R, et al.: Neonatal radiocontrast nephropathy simulating infantile polycystic kidney disease. Pediatrics 100:85, 1982.

Martin B, Conte J: Ultrasonography of the acute scrotum. J Clin Ultrasound 15:37, 1987.

Orazi C, Fariello G, Malena S, et al.: Torsion of paradidymis or Giraldes' organ: An uncommon cause of acute scrotum in pediatric age group. J Clin Ultrasound 17:598, 1989.

Testes

ABNORMAL ECHOGENICITY

Common

	Comment
Seminoma	Hypoechoic; well-circumscribed in 40% to 50% of tumors
Embryonal cell carcinoma	Hypoechoic, well-circumscribed; less homogeneous than seminomas
Choriocarcinoma	Complex mass; may have calcium
Mixed germ cell lesions	Inhomogeneous mass
Lymphoma	More common with non-Hodgkin's; may be focal or diffusely hypoechoic
Leukemia	May be focal or diffusely hypoechoic

Uncommon

Teratocarcinoma	Complex mass; may have calcification
Teratoma	
Epidermoid cyst	
Torsion	May rarely give generalized increase in echogenicity; more often echogenicity is decreased
Metastases	Especially lung, prostate, and GI tumors
Epididymal tumors	
Hematoma	
Abscess	More often in diabetics
Infarcts	May be focal or diffusely hypoechoic
Leydig's cell tumors	
Lipomas	
Sertoli's cell tumors	
Sarcoidosis	Hypoechoic; multiple
Adrenal rests	
Postsurgical defects	
Tunica albuginea cysts	
Brucellosis	Epididymis usually enlarged also; testicle inhomogeneous

Uncommon (Continued)	*Comment*
Myeloma of testicle	
Plasmacytoma	
Focal orchitis	Hyperechoic; adjacent to large epididymis
Malacoplakia	Diffuse or focal areas of decreased echogenicity
Lipoma	Echogenic focus within testes
Fibrosis	Hyperechoic
Adenomatoid tumor	Hyperechoic

Benson CB, Deligdish CK, Loughlin KR: Sonographic detection of testicular plasmacytoma. J Clin Ultrasound 15:490, 1987.

Burke BJ, Parker SH, Hopper KD, et al.: The ultrasonographic appearance of coexistent epididymal and testicular sarcoidosis. J Clin Ultrasound 18:522, 1990.

Chinn DH, Miller EI: Generalized testicular hyperechogenicity in acute testicular torsion. J Ultrasound Med 4:495, 1985.

Gale JT, Bowie JD, Mahony BS: Myeloma of the testicle: Sonographic appearance. J Clin Ultrasound 15:280, 1987.

Goodman A, Lipinski JK: Sonographic findings in malacoplakia of the testis with pathologic review. J Clin Ultrasound 12:45, 1984.

Kravitz JR, Ridlen MS: Imaging of an oat cell metastasis to the testicle: Case report and review of the literature. J Clin Ultrasound 18:121, 1990.

Lentini JF, Benson CB, Richie JP: Sonographic features of focal orchitis. J Ultrasound Med 8:361, 1989.

Martin B, Conte J: Ultrasonography of the acute scrotum. J Clin Ultrasound 15:37, 1987.

Maxwell AJ, Mamtora H: Sonographic appearance of epidermoid cyst of the testis. J Clin Ultrasound 18:188, 1990.

Patel PJ, Kolawole TM, Sharma N, et al.: Sonographic findings in scrotal brucellosis. J Clin Ultrasound 16:483, 1988.

Rosenberg R, Williamson MR: Lipomas of the spermatic cord and testis: Report of two cases. J Clin Ultrasound 17:670, 1989.

Vick CW, Bird KI, Jr., Rosenfield AT, Taylor KJW: Scrotal masses with a uniformly hyperechoic pattern. Radiology 148:209, 1983.

ENLARGED TESTICLE

Common	Comment
Tumors	Intrinsic tumors of testes
After trauma	May be edematous

Uncommon

Idiopathic macroorchidism
Brucellosis
Metastatic lymphoproliferative disease
Myeloma of testicle

Gale JT, Bowie JD, Mahony BS: Myeloma of the testicle: Sonographic appearance. J Clin Ultrasound 15:280, 1987.

Martin B, Conte J: Ultrasonography of the acute scrotum. J Clin Ultrasound 15:37, 1987.

Patel PJ, Kolawole TM, Sharma N, et al.: Sonographic findings in scrotal brucellosis. J Clin Ultrasound 16:483, 1988.

Phillips G, Kumari-Subaiya S, Sawitsky A: Ultrasonic evaluation of the scrotum in lymphoproliferative disease. J Ultrasound Med 6:169, 1987.

Truwit CL, Jackson M, Thompson IM: Idiopathic macroorchidism. J Clin Ultrasound 17:200, 1989.

CYSTS

	Comment
Cystic testicular tumor	Form from spermatic ducts
Cyst of tunica albuginea	
Benign non-neoplastic cyst	

Hamm B, Fobbe F, Loy V: Testicular cysts: Differentiation with US and clinical findings. Radiology 168:19, 1988.

ENLARGED EPIDIDYMIS

Common   *Comment*

Epididymitis
Sperm granuloma
Adenomatoid tumor

Uncommon

Brucellosis   Testicle has abnormal echogenicity
Sarcoidosis
Carcinoid tumor
Papillary cystadenoma
Leiomyoma
Fibroma
Adrenal rest
Cholesteatoma
Lipoma
Polyorchidism

Forte MD, Brant WE: Ultrasonographic detection of epididymal sarcoidosis. J Clin Ultrasound 16:191, 1988.
Patel PJ, Kolawole TM, Sharma N, et al.: Sonographic findings in scrotal brucellosis. J Clin Ultrasound 16:483, 1988.
Ramanathan K, Yaghoobian J, Pinck RL: Sperm granuloma. J Clin Ultrasound 14:155, 1986.

CALCIFICATION

With cryptorchidism
Klinefelter's syndrome
With testicular tumors
With pulmonary alveolar microlithiasis
Epidermoid cyst
TB
Granulomatous orchitis
Old hematoma
Phlebolith in varicocele

Bieger RC, Passarage E, McAdams AJ: Testicular intratubular bodies. J Clin Endocrinol Metab 25:1340, 1965.
Coetzee T: Pulmonary alveolar microlithiasis with involvement of the sympathetic nervous system and gonads. Thorax 25:637, 1970.
Doherty FJ, Mullins TL, Sant GR, et al.: Testicular microlithiasis: A unique sonographic appearance. J Ultrasound Med 6:389, 1987.

Gottlieb RH, Poster R, Subudhi MK: Computed tomographic, ultrasound, and plain film appearance of phleboliths in varicoceles. J Ultrasound Med 8:239, 1989.

Lanman JT, Sklarkin BS, Cooper HL, et al.: Klinefelter's syndrome in a ten-month-old Mongolian idiot: Report of a case with chromosome analysis. N Engl J Med 263:887, 1960.

Martin B, Tubiana JM: Significance of scrotal calcifications detected by sonography. J Clin Ultrasound 16:545, 1988.

Nistal M, Paniagua R, Diez-Pardo JA: Testicular microlithiasis in 2 children with bilateral cryptorchidism. J Urol 121:535, 1979.

Vegni-Talluri M, Bigliardi E, Vanni MG, et al.: Testicular microliths: Their origin and structure. J Urol 124:105, 1980.

HYPOECHOIC BANDS

Normal mediastinum testis
Normal vessels

Fakhry J, Khoury A, Barakat K: The hypoechoic band: A normal finding on testicular sonography. AJR 153:321, 1989.

Prostate

CYSTS

Common

Comment

Seminal vesicle cysts
In prostatitis
With benign prostatic hypertrophy
  (BPH)

Uncommon

Müllerian duct cysts   Originates at verumontanum
Utricle cysts   In juveniles and children
Abscess
Hydroureter
Cystocele
Parasitic cysts
With carcinoma

Eisenberg D, Luis-Jorge JC, Himmelfarb EH, et al.: Sonographic diagnosis of seminal vesicle cysts. J
  Clin Ultrasound 14:213, 1986.
Francis RA, Lewis E: Ultrasonic demonstration of a Müllerian duct cyst. J Ultrasound Med 2:525,
  1983.
Hamilton S, Fitzpatrick JM: Ultrasound diagnosis of a prostatic cyst causing acute urinary retention. J
  Ultrasound Med 6:385, 1987.
Hamper UM, Epstein JI, Sheth S, et al.: Cystic lesions of the prostate gland: A sonographic-pathologic
  correlation. J Ultrasound Med 9:395, 1990.

HYPOECHOIC LESIONS

Common	Comment
Cancer	
BPH	
Prostatitis	

Uncommon	
Malacoplakia	Granulomatous infection
Cysts	See preceding category
Abscess	

Chantelois AE, Parker SH, Sims JE, et al.: Malacoplakia of the prostate sonographically mimicking carcinoma. Radiology 177:193, 1990.

Lee F, Gray GM, McLeary RD, et al.: Prostatic evaluation by transrectal sonography: Criteria for diagnosis of early carcinoma. Radiology 158:91, 1986.

CALCIFICATIONS

Common	Comment
Calcified corpora amylacea	Coarse

Uncommon	
Necrotic tumor	Fine, stippled
Benign tumors	

Hamper UM, Sheth S, Walsh PC, et al.: Bright echogenic foci in early prostatic carcinoma: Sonographic and pathologic correlation. Radiology 176:339, 1990.

ECHOGENIC LESION

Common   Comment

BPH
Corpora amylacea

Uncommon

Cancer   Occasionally echogenic
Foreign body in urethra   Catheter is most common
Calcifications

Fornage BD: Transrectal ultrasound diagnosis of a misplaced Foley catheter. J Clin Ultrasound 14:629, 1986.

Hamper UM, Sheth S, Walsh PC, et al.: Bright echogenic foci in early prostatic carcinoma: Sonographic and pathologic correlation. Radiology 176:339, 1990.

SEMINAL VESICLE ABNORMALITIES

Common

Cysts
Extension of prostate cancer

Leiomyomas
Adenocarcinoma
Cystadenoma
Angiosarcoma

Bahn DK, Brown RKJ, Shei KY, et al.: Sonographic findings of leiomyoma in the seminal vesicle. J Clin Ultrasound 18:517, 1990.

Bullock KN: Cystadenoma of the seminal vesicle. J R Soc Med 81(5):294, 1988.

Davis NS, Merguerian PA, DiMarco PL, et al.: Primary adenocarcinoma of seminal vesicle presenting as bladder carcinoma. Urology 32(5):466, 1988.

Eisenberg D, Luis-Jorge JC, Himmelfarb EH, et al.: Sonographic diagnosis of seminal vesicle cysts. J Clin Ultrasound 14:213, 1986.

Panageas E, Kuligowska E, Dunlop R, et al.: Angiosarcoma of the seminal vesicle: Early detection using transrectal ultrasound-guided biopsy. J Clin Ultrasound 18:666, 1990.

Tanaka T, Takeuchi T, Oguchi K, et al.: Primary adenocarcinoma of the seminal vesicle. Hum Pathol 18(2):200, 1987.

PART II
OBSTETRICS

FETAL HEAD AND FACE

Hydrocephalus
Pericranial mass
Cystic mass within cranium
Small cranium
Increased ventricular separation
Intracranial tumors
Cloverleaf skull (Kleeblattschädel)
  syndrome
Absence of calvarium
Hypotelorism
Hypertelorism

FETAL HEAD AND NECK

Low-set ears
Neck masses
Cystic hygromas
Nuchal skin thickening
Microphthalmia (small orbital
  diameter)
Proboscis
Macroglossia
Cleft lip and palate

FETAL THORAX

Pleural effusion
Lung mass
Mediastinal mass

FETAL HEART

Cardiomegaly
Overriding aorta
Fluid around heart
Heart tumors
Ectopia cordis
Arrhythmias
Shift of heart
Defect in atrial septum
Defect in ventricular septum
Atrioventricular septal defects
Single ventricle
Large right atrium
Small left ventricle
Small right ventricle
Enlarged right ventricle
Enlarged left ventricle
Thickened left ventricle wall
Thickened right ventricle wall
Enlarged pulmonary artery
Small pulmonary artery
Small aorta
Enlarged aorta
Small left atrium

FETAL ABDOMEN

Anterior abdominal wall defects or
  masses
Nonvisualization of stomach
Fetal stomach mass
Double bubble
Dilated loops of bowel

Abdominal cysts
Abdominal mass

FETAL LIVER

Hepatomegaly

FETAL SPLEEN

Splenomegaly
Small or hypoplastic spleen

FETAL ASCITES (BY ETIOLOGY)

Hematologic
Pulmonary
Neurologic
Gastrointestinal
Hepatic
Genitourinary
Infectious
Neoplastic
Cardiovascular
Metabolic
Skeletal
Trisomies
Hereditary
Placental

FETAL ADRENALS

Masses

FETAL KIDNEYS

Enlarged kidneys
Cysts in kidneys
Echogenic kidneys
Hydronephrosis
Empty renal fossa

FETAL BLADDER

Nonvisualization of bladder
Distended bladder

FETAL PELVIS

Masses

FETAL SKELETON

Skeletal dysplasias
Decreased ossification, calvarium
Multiple contractures
Clubfoot
Widened metaphyses
Bone demineralization
Joint laxity/dislocation
Polydactyly
Clavicular hypoplasia
Absence of limb or segment
 of limb
Enlarged limb
Rocker-bottom feet

FLUID ABNORMALITIES

Polyhydramnios
Oligohydramnios
Nonimmune hydrops fetalis

CORD AND PLACENTA

Umbilical cord masses
Placental lucencies
Placental masses
Enlarged (thickened) placenta

FETAL SIZE

Large for dates

INTRAUTERINE MEMBRANES

Fetal Head and Face

HYDROCEPHALUS

	Comment
Communicating	Obstruction outside ventricles
Aqueductal stenosis	Fourth ventricle is normal
Dandy-Walker syndrome	Post fossa cyst
Arnold-Chiari II syndrome (associated with spina bifida)	Obstruction outside ventricles
Choroid plexus papilloma	Mass in ventricle
Hydranencephaly	
Lobar holoprosencephaly	Ventricles splayed apart
Triploidy	

Hashimoto BE, Mahoney BS, Fify RA, et al.: Sonography, a complementary examination to alpha fetoprotein testing for fetal neural tube defects. J Ultrasound Med 4:307, 1985.

Nyberg DA, Cyr DR, Mack LA, et al.: The Dandy-Walker malformation prenatal sonographic diagnosis and its clinical significance. J Ultrasound Med 7:65, 1988.

Pilu G, De Palma L, Romero R, et al.: The fetal subarachnoid cisterns: An ultrasound study with report of a case of congenital communicating hydrocephalus. J Ultrasound Med 5:365, 1986.

PERICRANIAL MASS

	Comment
Normal fetal hair	Seen after 24 weeks
Hemangioma	
Cephaloceles	May see brain tissue within
Cystic hygromas	Usually septa
Scalp edema	
Cephalohematoma	
Subcutaneous hematoma	

Chervenak FA, Isaacson G, Mahoney MJ, et al.: Diagnosis and management of fetal cephalocele. Obstet Gynecol 64:86, 1984.

Grylack L: Prenatal sonographic diagnosis of cephalohematoma due to prelabor trauma. Pediatr Radiol 12:145, 1982.

Harper AK, Clark JA, Koontz WL, et al.: Sonographic appearance of fetal extracranial hematoma. J Ultrasound Med 8:693, 1989.

Petrikovsky BM, Vintzileos AM, Rodis JF: Sonographic appearance of occipital fetal hair. J Clin Ultrasound 17:425, 1989.

CYSTIC MASS WITHIN CRANIUM

	Comment
Dandy-Walker cyst	Associated with vermis hypoplasia
Porencephaly	May have asymmetric vents
Schizencephaly	Migration failure
Arachnoid cyst	
Cystic tumor	
Hydranencephaly	No cortex; no midline echo
Holoprosencephaly	Alobar with no interhemispheric fissure
Choroid plexus cyst	
Vein of Galen aneurysm	Doppler shows high flow
After in utero hemorrhage	May occur in neonatal thrombocytopenia
Subdural hygroma	

Benacerraf BR: Asymptomatic cysts of the fetal choroid plexus in the second trimester. J Ultrasound Med 6:475, 1987.

Body G, Darnis E, Pourcelot D, et al.: Choroid plexus tumors: Antenatal diagnosis and follow-up. J Clin Ultrasound 18:575, 1990.

Carrasco CR, Stierman ED, Harnsberger HR, et al.: An algorithm for prenatal ultrasound diagnosis of congenital central nervous system abnormalities. J Ultrasound Med 4:163, 1985.

Fakhry J, Schechter A, Tenner MS, et al.: Cysts of the choroid plexus in neonates: Documentation and review of the literature. J Ultrasound Med 4:561, 1985.

Filly RA, Chinn DH, Callen PW: Alobar holoprosencephaly: Ultrasonographic prenatal diagnosis. Radiology 151:455, 1984.

Fiske CE, Filly RA: Ultrasound evaluation of the normal and abnormal fetal neural axis. Radiol Clin North Am 20:285, 1982.

Ghidini A, Vergani P, Sirtori M, et al.: Prenatal diagnosis of subdural hygroma. J Ultrasound Med 7:463, 1988.

Hertzberg BS, Kay HH, Bowie JD: Fetal choroid plexus lesions: Relationship of antenatal sonographic appearance to clinical outcome. J Ultrasound Med 8:77, 1989.

Hoffman-Tretin JC, Horoupian DS, Loenigsberg M, et al.: Lobar holoprosencephaly with hydrocephalus: Antenatal demonstration and differential diagnosis. J Ultrasound Med 5:691, 1986.

Komarniske CA, Cyr DR, Mack LA, et al.: Prenatal diagnosis of schizencephaly. J Ultrasound Med 9:305, 1990.

Lester RB, Sty JR: Prenatal diagnosis of cystic CNS lesions in neonatal isoimmune thrombocytopenia. J Ultrasound Med 6:479, 1987.

Meizner I, Barki Y, Tadmor R, et al.: In utero ultrasonic detection of fetal arachnoid cyst. J Clin Ultrasound 16:506, 1988.

Nyberg DA, Cyr DR, Mack LA, et al.: The Dandy-Walker malformation prenatal sonographic diagnosis and its clinical significance. J Ultrasound Med 7:65, 1988.

Sauerbrei EE, Cooperberg PL: Cystic tumors of the fetal and neonatal cerebrum: Ultrasound and computed tomographic evaluation. Radiology 147:689, 1983.

Shawker TH, Schwartz RM: Ultrasound appearance of a malignant fetal brain tumor. J Clin Ultrasound 11:35, 1983.

SMALL CRANIUM

Comment

Off dates
Symmetric intrauterine growth
   retardation (IUGR)
Microcephaly   Has sloping forehead
Craniosynostosis

Pearce JM, Little D, Campbell S: The diagnosis of abnormalities of the fetal central nervous system, in Sanders RC, James EA (eds): *The Principles and Practice of Ultrasonography in Obstetrics and Gynecology*, 3d ed. Norwalk, Conn, Appleton-Century-Crofts, 1985, pp 243-256.

INCREASED VENTRICULAR SEPARATION

Comment

Agenesis of corpus callosum   Enlarged atria
Lobar holoprosencephaly

INTRACRANIAL TUMORS

Comment

Embryonic tumors
  Epidermoid
  Dermoid
  Teratoma   Cystic and solid appearance
Germinal tumors
  Germinoma
  Embryonal carcinoma
  Choriocarcinoma
  Endodermal sinus tumor
  Teratoma
Neuroblastic tumors
  Medulloblastoma
  Neuroblastoma
  Retinoblastoma
Embryonal remnant tumors
  Craniopharyngioma   Complex mass
  Chordoma
Ependymal origin
  Ependymoma
  Subependymal mixed glioma
  Choroid plexus papilloma
  Glioblastoma multiforme
  Malignant astrocytoma
  Choroid plexus cysts
Associated with genetic diseases
  Tuberous sclerosis
  Neurofibromatosis
  Systemic angiomatosis (von Hipple-
    Lindau)
Colloid cyst of third ventricle
Heterotopia and hamartoma
Lipoma   Common in corpus callosum
Vascular tumors: hemangioblastoma
Intracranial hemorrhage
Pseudoepidural artifact   Reverberations from distal cranial bone
Dandy-Walker cyst

Benacerraf BR: Asymptomatic cysts of the fetal choroid plexus in the second trimester. J Ultrasound Med 6:475, 1987.

Body G, Darnis E, Pourcelot D, et al.: Choroid plexus tumors: Antenatal diagnosis and follow-up. J Clin Ultrasound 18:575, 1990.

Christensen RA, Pinckney LE, Higgins S, et al.: Sonographic diagnosis of lipoma of the corpus callosum. J Ultrasound Med 6:449, 1987.

Crade M: Ultrasonic demonstration in utero of an intracranial teratoma. JAMA 247:1173, 1982.

Hoff NR, Mackay IM: Prenatal ultrasound diagnosis of intracranial teratoma. J Clin Ultrasound 8:247, 1980.

Kirkinen P, Suramo I, Jouppila P, et al.: Combined use of ultrasound and computed tomography in the evaluation of fetal intracranial abnormality. J Perinat Med 10:257, 1982.

Mintz MC, Arger PH, Coleman BG: In utero sonographic diagnosis of intracerebral hemorrhage. J Ultrasound Med 4:375, 1985.

Nyberg DA, Cyr DR, Mack LA, et al.: The Dandy-Walker malformation prenatal sonographic diagnosis and its clinical significance. J Ultrasound Med 7:65, 1988.

Ostlere SJ, Irving HC, Lilford RJ: Fetal choroid plexus cysts: A report of 100 cases. Radiology 175:753, 1990.

Snyder JR, Lustig-Gillman I, Milio L, et al.: Antenatal ultrasound diagnosis of an intracranial neoplasm (craniopharyngioma). J Clin Ultrasound 14:304, 1986.

Stanley JH, Harrell B, Horger EO: Pseudoepidural reverberation artifact: A common ultrasound artifact in fetal cranium. J Clin Ultrasound 14:251, 1986.

Vinters HV, Murphy J, Wittman B, et al.: Intracranial teratoma: Antenatal diagnosis at 31 weeks gestation by ultrasound. Acta Neuropathol 58:233, 1982.

Wilson CB et al.: Pathology of intercranial tumors, in Newton TH, Potts DG (eds): *Radiology of the Skull and Brain. Anatomy and Pathology.* St. Louis, CV Mosby, 1977.

CLOVERLEAF SKULL (KLEEBLATTSCHÄDEL) SYNDROME

	Comment
With thanatophoric dysplasia	Autosomal recessive
Craniosynostosis	
Amniotic bands	

Cohen MM: Genetic perspectives on craniosynostosis in syndromes with craniosynostosis. J Neurosurg 47:886, 1977.

Stamm ER, Pretorius DH, Rumack CM, et al.: Kleeblattschädel anomaly: In utero sonographic appearance. J Ultrasound Med 6:319, 1987.

Weiner CP, Williamson RA, Bonsib SM: Sonographic diagnosis of cloverleaf skull and thanatophoric dysplasia in the second trimester. J Clin Ultrasound 14:463, 1986.

ABSENCE OF CALVARIUM

Acrania
Anencephaly
Encephaloceles
Lack of skull mineralization

Mannes EJ, Crelin ES, Hobbins JC, et al.: Sonographic demonstration of fetal acrania. AJR 139:181, 1982.

HYPOTELORISM

Holoprosencephaly
Trigonocephaly
Oculodentodigital dysplasia
Microcephaly
Meckel's syndrome
Maternal phenylketonuria
Chromosomal aberrations
Trisomy 13
Trisomy 21
18p −
5p −
14q +

Romero R, Pilu G, Jeanty P, Ghidini A, Hobbins J: *Prenatal Diagnosis of Congenital Anomalies.* Norwalk, Conn, Appleton & Lange, 1988, p 96.

HYPERTELORISM*

Comment

With other median plane facial
  malformations
  Median-cleft-face syndrome
  Frontal, ethmoidal, or sphenoidal
    meningoencephalocele
  Frontal, ethmoidal, or sphenoidal
    dermo-lipoma-teratoma
  Nasal glioma
  Nasofrontal mucoceles
With miscellaneous facial defects
  Proboscis lateralis
  Facial clefts other than median
  Facial hemangioma
  Extra nares
With other skull dysplasias
  Craniosynostosis
  Apert's syndrome
  Crouzon's disease
  Pfeiffer's syndrome
  Carpenter's syndrome
  Kleeblattschädel syndrome
Thickened skull
  Albers-Schönberg disease
  Pyle's disease (craniometaphyseal
    dysplasia)
Metopism
With teeth defects: Rieger's syndrome
With prominent brain/neurological
  defects
  Hydrocephalus (any type)
  Megaloencephaly with skull
    enlargement
  Familial neurovisceral lipidosis
  Lissencephaly
  Agenesis of septum pellucidum
  Agenesis of corpus callosum
With ocular defects
With cleft/lip palate
With prominent skin manifestations
With prominent skeletal malformations
With sexual organ malformations
With chromosomal abnormalities

* Adapted from Romero et al. (1988).

HYPERTELORISM (Continued)

Comment

Miscellaneous
   Hypercalcemia with supravalvular
      aortic stenosis
   Potter's syndrome
   With inguinal hernia
   Lymphedema and yellow nails
   AIDS dysmorphism
   Noonan's syndrome   Cystic hygromas; renal and cardiac
                                        anomalies

Benacerraf BR, Greene MF, Holmes LB: The prenatal sonographic features of Noonan's syndrome. J
   Ultrasound Med 8:59, 1989.
Romero R, Pilu G, Jeanty P, Ghidini A, Hobbins J: *Prenatal Diagnosis of Congenital Anomalies.*
   Norwalk, Conn, Appleton & Lange, 1988, pp 90-91.

Fetal Head and Neck

LOW-SET EARS

	Comment
Otocephaly	Hypoplasia of mandible and proximity of temporal bones
Treacher Collins syndrome	

Cayea PD, Bieber FR, Ross MJ, et al.: Sonographic findings in otocephaly (synotia). J Ultrasound Med 4:377, 1985.

NECK MASSES

Common

	Comment
Cystic hygroma	Multiseptate
Nonimmune hydrops	

Uncommon

	Comment
Cervical meningocele	
Cephalocele	Bony defect in skull
Neck tumors	Usually complex
Klippel-Trenaunay-Weber syndrome	Have cutaneous hemangiomas
Subcutaneous edema	
Goiter	Solid mass; head hyperextended
Brachial cleft cyst	Purely cystic
Hemangioma	Cystic or solid
Teratomas	Usually complex
Neuroblastoma of neck	40% to 45% calcified
Hemangioendothelioma	Solid
Twin sac of blighted ovum	
Nuchal bleb	

Barone CM, Van Natta FC, Kourides IA, et al.: Sonographic detection of fetal goiter, an unusual cause of hydramnios. J Ultrasound Med 4:625, 1985.

Bieber FR, Petres RE, Bieber J, et al.: Prenatal detection of a familial nuchal bleb simulating encephalocele. Birth Defects XV(5A):51, 1979.

Byrne J, Blanc WA, Warburton D, et al.: The significance of cystic hygroma in fetuses. Hum Pathol 15:61, 1984.

Chervenak FA, Isaacson G, Blakemore KJ, et al.: Fetal cystic hygroma. Cause and natural history. N Engl J Med 309:822, 1983.

Chervenak FA, Isaacson G, Torotra M: A sonographic study of fetal cystic hygromas. J Clin Ultrasound 13:311, 1985.

Gadwood KA, Reynes CJ: Prenatal sonography of metastatic neuroblastoma of the neck. J Clin Ultrasound 11:512, 1983.

Kourides IA, Berkowitz RL, Pang S, et al.: Antepartum diagnosis of goitrous hypothyroidism by fetal ultrasonography and amniotic fluid thyrotropin concentration. J Clin Endocrinol Metab 59:1016, 1984.

McGahan JP, Schneider JM: Fetal neck hemangioendothelioma with secondary hydrops fetalis: Sonographic diagnosis. J Clin Ultrasound 14:384, 1986.

Pearce JM, Griffin D, Campbell S: The differential prenatal diagnosis of cystic hygromata and encephalocele by ultrasound examination. J Clin Ultrasound 13:317, 1985.

Rosenfeld CR, Coln CD, Duenhoelter JH: Fetal cervical teratoma as a cause of polyhydramnios. Pediatrics 64:176, 1979.

Shalev E, Romano S, Nseir T, et al.: Klippel-Trenaunay syndrome: Ultrasonic prenatal diagnosis. J Clin Ultrasound 16:268, 1988.

Trecet JC, Claramunt V, Larraz J, et al.: Prenatal U/S diagnosis of fetal teratoma of the neck. J Clin Ultrasound 12:509, 1984.

CYSTIC HYGROMAS

Common	Comment
Turner's syndrome	
Trisomy 21	

Uncommon	
Noonan's syndrome	Hypertelorism; renal anomalies; short stature; heart anomalies
Distichiasis-lymphedema syndrome	
Multiple pterygium syndrome	Pterygia of neck, axillae, elbows, knees; micrognathia; camptodactylia; syndactylia; rocker-bottom feet
Robert's syndrome	
Lethal nuchal cyst syndrome	

Benacerraf BR, Greene MF, Holmes LB: The prenatal sonographic features of Noonan's syndrome. J Ultrasound Med 8:59, 1989.

Benacerraf BR, Saltzman DH, Sanders SP: Sonographic sign suggesting the prenatal diagnosis of coarctation of the aorta. J Ultrasound Med 8:65, 1989.

Chervenak FA, Isaacson G, Blakemore KJ, et al.: Fetal cystic hygroma: Cause and natural history. N Engl J Med 309:822, 1983.

Elejalde BR, Mercedes de Elejalde M, Leno J: Nuchal cyst syndrome: Etiology, pathogenesis, and prenatal diagnosis. Am J Med Genet 21:417, 1985.

Garden AS, Benzie RJ, Miskin M, et al.: Fetal cystic hygroma colli: Antenatal diagnosis, significance, and management. Am J Obstet Gynecol 154:221, 1986.

Macken MB, Grantmyre EB, Vincer MJ: Regression of nuchal cystic hygroma in utero. J Ultrasound Med 8:101, 1989.

Pearce JM, Griffin D, Campbell S: The differential prenatal diagnosis of cystic hygromata and encephalocele by ultrasound examination. J Clin Ultrasound 13:317, 1985.

Zarabi M, Mieckowski GC, Mazer J: Cystic hygroma associated with Noonan's syndrome. J Clin Ultrasound 11:398, 1983.

NUCHAL SKIN THICKENING

	Comment
Trisomy 21	>5 mm between 15 to 20 wks
13q syndrome	
XXXX syndrome	
XXXXY syndrome	
Trisomy 18	
18p− syndrome	
Multiple pterygium syndrome	Pterygia of neck, axillae, elbows, knees; micrognathia; camptodactylia; syndactylia; rocker-bottom feet
Klippel-Feil syndrome	Fusion of cervical vertebrae; ventricular septal defect (VSD)
Zellweger syndrome	Large forehead; flat facies; cystic kidneys; micrognathia
Normal specular reflector	

Benacerraf BR, Barss VA, Laboda LA: A sonographic sign for the detection in the second trimester of the fetus with Down's syndrome. Am J Obstet Gynecol 151:1078, 1985.

Benacerraf BR, Frigoletto FD, Laboda LA: Sonographic diagnosis of Down syndrome in the second trimester. Am J Obstet Gynecol 153:49, 1985.

Escobar V, Bixler D, Gleiser S, et al.: Multiple pterygium syndrome. Am J Dis Child 132:609, 1978.

Hertzberg BS, Bowie JD, Carroll BS, et al.: Normal sonographic appearance of the fetal neck late in the first trimester: The pseudomembrane. Radiology 171:427, 1989.

Toi A, Simpson GF, Filly RA: Ultrasonically evident fetal nuchal skin thickening: Is it specific for Down syndrome? Am J Obstet Gynecol 156:150, 1987.

MICROPHTHALMIA (SMALL ORBITAL DIAMETER)

	Comment
Some normals	
Chromosomal abnormalities	
Fetal toxoplasmosis	Hydrocephalus; splenomegaly; nonimmune hydrops
Fetal rubella	Hepatosplenomegaly; cardiac defects
Fetal alcohol syndrome	Scoliosis and skeletal anomalies, microcephaly and neural tube defects, and genitourinary (GU) anomalies
Fetal varicella	Hydrocephalus; gastrointestinal (GI) and GU anomalies
Maternal phenylketonuria	
CHARGE association	Coloboma (eye), heart disease, choanal atresia, retarded growth and development (with or without CNS anomalies), genital hypoplasia, ear anomalies (with or without deafness); two or more needed to make the diagnosis
Frontonasal dysplasia (median cleft face)	
Fraser's syndrome	GU anomalies; syndactyly
Goldenhar-Gorlin syndrome	Hypoplasia of mandible, maxilla, and temporal bones; vertebral anomalies; brain abnormalities
Lenz's syndrome	GU anomalies; scoliosis; GI anomalies
Goltz syndrome	Syndactyly; microcephaly; scoliosis
Hallermann-Streiff syndrome	Brachycephaly; small face; gracile tubular bones; vertebral anomalies
Oculodentodigital syndrome	Syndactyly
Pena-Shokeir II syndrome	Renal anomalies; hip dislocation
Fanconi's syndrome	Dwarfism and ricketts

Romero R, Pilu G, Jeanty P, Ghidini A, Hobbins J: *Prenatal Diagnosis of Congenital Anomalies.* Norwalk, Conn, Appleton & Lange, 1988, p 98.

PROBOSCIS

Holoprosencephaly
Chromosomal anomalies

MACROGLOSSIA

Comment

Beckwith-Wiedemann syndrome　　Omphalocele; organomegaly
Tumor of tongue

Koontz WL, Shaw LA, Lavery JP: Antenatal sonographic appearance of Beckwith-Wiedemann syndrome. J Clin Ultrasound 14:57, 1986.

CLEFT LIP AND PALATE

Autosomal Dominant Cleft Syndromes*

	Comment
Cleft lip or palate or both and lip pits	Van der Woude's syndrome
Cleft lip or palate or both and ankyloblepharon filiforme adnatum	
Cleft lip/palate, lobster-claw deformity, dacryocystitis, and hypodontia	Most sporadic cases
Cleft lip or palate or both and enlarged parietal foramina	Uncertain
Cleft lip or palate or both and congenital neuroblastoma	
Cleft lip or palate or both and popliteal pterygia	
Cleft palate and hereditary arthroophthalmopathy	
Cleft palate, retinal detachment, and myopia	
Cleft palate, retinal detachment, and joint hypermobility	
Cleft lip or palate or both and multiple nevoid basal cell carcinoma	
Cleft palate and the Apert's syndrome	
Cleft palate and the Marfan's syndrome	
Cleft lip or palate or both and Waardenburg's syndrome	
Cleft palate and mandibulofacial dysostosis	
Cleft palate and congenital spondyloepiphyseal dysplasia	
Cleft lip/palate, hypohidrosis, thin wiry hair, and dystrophic nails	
Cleft palate, camptodactyly, and clubfoot	

*Adapted from Romero et al. (1988).

CLEFT LIP AND PALATE (Continued)

Autosomal Dominant Cleft Syndromes*

	Comment
Cleft lip/palate, tetraphocomelia, and penile or clitoral enlargement	
Cleft lip/palate and pseudo-thalidomide syndrome	
Cleft palate and Klippel-Feil syndrome	Genetic pattern uncertain
Cleft palate and chondrodysplasia punctata	
Cleft palate and multiple congenital dislocations	Larsen's syndrome
Cleft palate and diastrophic dwarfism	
Cleft palate and the Smith-Lemli-Opitz syndrome	
Cleft palate and the Meckel's syndrome	
Cleft palate and the multiple pterygium syndrome	

CLEFT LIP AND PALATE (Continued)

X-Linked Cleft Syndromes

	Comment
Otopalatodigital syndrome	Probably X-linked recessive (XLR)
Orofaciodigital syndrome I	X-linked dominant (XLD); lethal in males
Cleft uvula, familial nephrons, deafness, congenital urinary trace, and digital anomalies	XLR
Cleft lip or palate or both and cryptophthalmos syndrome	Fraser's syndrome
Cleft lip/palate, ocular hypertelorism, and microtia	
Cleft lip/palate, microcephaly, and hypoplasia of radii and thumbs	
Cleft lip/palate, tetraperomelia, deformed pinna, and ectodermal dysplasia	
Cleft palate, stapes fixation, and oligodontia	
Cleft palate and cerebrocosto-mandibular syndrome	
Cleft palate and orofaciodigital syndrome II	
Cleft palate and new chondrodysplasia	
Cleft palate, median cleft lip, and unknown lethal chondrodysplasia	

CLEFT LIP AND PALATE (Continued)

Nongenetic Cleft Syndromes

	Comment
Robin's syndrome	Rare familial occurrence
Cleft lip/palate and cleft larynx	
Cleft lip/palate and laryngeal web	
Cleft lip or palate or both and thoracopagus twins	
Facial clefts and amniotic band syndrome	
Cleft lip or palate or both and forearm bone aplasia	
Cleft lip or palate or both and congenital heart disease	
Cleft lip or palate or both and anencephaly	
Cleft palate and Brachmann-de Lange syndrome	
Cleft palate and glossopalatine ankylosis	
Cleft lip/palate and lateral proboscis	
Premaxillary agenesis	May also occur with trisomy 13 and 18p −
Cleft lip or palate or both and encephalomeningocele	
Cleft lip or palate or both and median cleft face syndrome	
Cleft palate and congenital oral teratoma	
Cleft palate and buccopharyngeal membrane persistence	
Cleft palate and oral duplication	
Cleft palate and bilateral femoral dysplasia	
Oromandibular limb hypogenesis	

CLEFT LIP AND PALATE (Continued)

Gross Chromosomal Cleft Syndromes

4p −
5p −
Trisomy C mosaicism
Trisomy 13
Dp −
14q −
Trisomy 18
18p −
18q −
Trisomy 21
XXXXY syndrome
Various translocations
Supernumerary G-sized fragments
Monosomy G
Triploidy

Romero R, Pilu G, Jeanty P, Ghidini A, Hobbins J: *Prenatal Diagnosis of Congenital Anomalies.* Norwalk, Conn, Appleton & Lange, 1988, p 102.

Shechter SA, Sherer DM, Geilfuss CJ, et al.: Prenatal sonographic appearance and subsequent management of a fetus with oromandibular limb hypogenesis syndrome associated with pulmonary hypoplasia. J Clin Ultrasound 18:661, 1990.

Fetal Thorax

PLEURAL EFFUSION

	Comment
Chylothorax	Usually right-sided
Pulmonary lymphangiectasia	
Tracheoesophageal fistula	
Extralobar lung sequestration	
Multiple anomalies	
Diaphragmatic hernia	
Nonimmune hydrops	
Enteric cyst	From duplication of foregut
Pena-Shokeir syndrome	Polyhydramnios; hydrops
Small fetal thorax	
Asphyxiating thoracic dystrophy	Also known as Jeune's syndrome
Pena-Shokeir syndrome	Polyhydramnios; hydrops
Cardiac failure	
Lymphatic obstruction at thoracic inlet	

Andersen EA, Hertel J, Pedersen SA, et al.: Congenital chylothorax: Management by ligature of the thoracic duct. Scand J Thorac Cardiovasc Surg 18:193, 1984.

Benacerraf BR, Frigoletto FD: Mid-trimester fetal thoracentesis. J Clin Ultrasound 13:202, 1985.

Callan NA, Colmorgen GC, Weiner S: Lung hypoplasia and prolonged preterm ruptured membranes: A case report with implications for possible prenatal ultrasonic diagnosis. Am J Obstet Gynecol 151:756, 1985.

Callan NA, Otis CS, Colmorgen GC, et al.: The ultrasonic measurement of normal fetal thoracic parameters: Implications in fetal compression, in Proceedings of the Society of Gynecological Investigation, San Francisco, 1984.

Cardwell MS: Pena-Shokeir syndrome: Prenatal diagnosis by ultrasonography. J Ultrasound Med 6:619, 1987.

Defoort P, Thiery M: Antenatal diagnosis of congenital chylothorax by gray scale sonography. J Clin Ultrasound 6:47, 1978.

Dresler S: Massive pleural effusion and hypoplasia of the lung accompanying extralobar pulmonary sequestration. Hum Pathol 12:862, 1981.

Franzek DA, Strayer SA, Hull MT, et al.: Enteric cyst as a cause of nonimmune hydrops fetalis: Fetal thoracentesis with fluid analysis. J Clin Ultrasound 17:275, 1989.

Harvey JG, Loulsby W, Sherman K, et al.: Congenital chylothorax: Report of unique case associated with "H"-type tracheo-oesophageal fistula. Br J Surg 66:485, 1979.

Hunter WS, Becroft DMQ: Congenital pulmonary lymphangiectasis associated with pleural effusions. Arch Dis Child 59:278, 1984.

Jaffa AJ, Barak S, Kaysar N, et al.: Case report. Antenatal diagnosis of bilateral congenital chylothorax with pericardial effusion. Acta Obstet Gynecol Scand 64:455, 1985.

Jouppila P, Kirkinen P, Herva R, et al.: Prenatal diagnosis of pleural effusions by ultrasound. J Clin Ultrasound 11:516, 1983.

Lange IR, Manning FA: Antenatal diagnosis of congenital pleural effusions. Am J Obstet Gynecol 140:839, 1981.

Lazarus KH, McCurdy FA: Multiple congenital anomalies in a patient with Diamond-Blackfan syndrome. Clin Pediatr 23:520, 1984.

Meizner I, Carmi R, Mares AJ, et al.: Spontaneous resolution of isolated fetal ascites associated with extralobar lung sequestration. J Clin Ultrasound 18:57, 1990.

Skiptunas SM, Weiner S: Early prenatal diagnosis of asphyxiating thoracic dysplasia (Jeune's syndrome): Value of fetal thoracic measurement. J Ultrasound Med 6:41, 1987.

Weiner C, Varner M, Pringle K, et al.: Antenatal diagnosis and palliative treatment of non-immune hydrops fetalis secondary to pulmonary extralobar sequestration. Obstet Gynecol 68:275, 1986.

LUNG MASS

	Comment
Cystic adenomatoid malformation	May be large cysts, small cysts, or solid mass
Diaphragmatic hernia	Look for peristalsis
Bronchogenic cysts	
Pulmonary sequestration	Solid lesion
Bronchopulmonary foregut malformation	Similar to sequestration
Bronchial atresia	
Teratomas	
Enteric cyst	From duplication of foregut
Rhabdomyoma	

Albright EB, Crane JP, Shackelford GD: Prenatal diagnosis of a bronchogenic cyst. J Ultrasound Med 7:91, 1988.

Buntain WL, Woolley MM, Mahour GH, et al.: Pulmonary sequestration in children: A twenty-five year experience. Surgery 81:413, 1977.

Cyr DR, Guntheroth WG, Nyberg DA, et al.: Prenatal diagnosis of an intrapericardial teratoma: A cause for nonimmune hydrops. J Ultrasound Med 7:87, 1988.

Demos NJ, Teresi A: Congenital lung malformations. A unified concept and a case report. J Thorac Cardiovasc Surg 70:260, 1975.

Franzek DA, Strayer SA, Hull MT, et al.: Enteric cyst as a cause of nonimmune hydrops fetalis: Fetal thoracentesis with fluid analysis. J Clin Ultrasound 17:275, 1989.

Goldblatt E, Vimpani G, Brown JH: Extralobar pulmonary sequestration. Presentation as an arteriovenous aneurysm with cardiac failure in infancy. Am J Cardiol 29:100, 1971.

Heithoff KB, Sane SM, Williams HJ, et al.: Bronchopulmonary foregut malformations. A unifying etiological concept. AJR 126:46, 1976.

Iwai K, Shindo G, Hajikano H, et al.: Intralobar pulmonary sequestration, with special reference to developmental pathology. Am Rev Respir Dis 107:911, 1973.

Knochel JQ, Lee TG, Melendez MG, et al.: Fetal anomalies involving the thorax and abdomen. Radiol Clin North Am 20:297, 1982.

Mariona F, McAlpin G, Zador I, et al.: Sonographic detection of fetal extrathoracic pulmonary sequestration. J Clin Ultrasound 5:283, 1986.

Mayden KL, Tortora M, Chervenak FA, et al.: The antenatal sonographic detection of lung masses. Am J Obstet Gynecol 148:349, 1984.

McAllister WH, Wright JR Jr., Crane JP: Main-stem bronchial atresia: Intrauterine sonographic diagnosis. AJR 148:364, 1987.

Pezzuti RT, Isler RJ: Antenatal ultrasound detection of cystic adenomatoid malformation of lung: Report of a case and review of the recent literature. J Clin Ultrasound 11:342, 1983.

Ramenofsky ML, Leape LL, McCauley RGK: Bronchogenic cyst. J Pediatr Surg 14:219, 1979.

Rempen A, Feige A, Wünsch P: Prenatal diagnosis of bilateral cystic adenomatoid malformation of the lung. J Clin Ultrasound 15:3, 1987.

Ryckman FC, Rosenkrantz JG: Thoracic surgical problems in infancy and childhood. Surg Clin North Am 65:1423, 1985.

Siffring P, Forrest TS, Hill WC, et al.: Prenatal sonographic diagnosis of bronchopulmonary foregut malformation. J Ultrasound Med 8:277, 1989.

MEDIASTINAL MASS

	Comment
Teratoma	Solid
Thymus or thymic neoplasm	Solid
Germ cell tumor	Solid
Goiter	Solid
Bronchogenic cyst	Cystic
Lymphangioma	Cystic
Hemangioma	Cystic
Pericardial cyst	Cystic
Diaphragmatic hernia	Cystic
Neurogenic tumor	Solid
Sequestration	Solid
Enteric cyst	Cystic
Esophageal duplication	Cystic
Anterior meningocele	Cystic
Neuroblastoma	Cystic
Bronchiectasis	Cystic
Mediastinal encephalocele	Cystic
Pericardial effusion	Cystic
Pleural effusion	Cystic

Albright EB, Crane JP, Shackelford GD: Prenatal diagnosis of a bronchogenic cyst. J Ultrasound Med 7:91, 1988.

Bower RJ, Kiesewetter WB: Mediastinal masses in infants and children. Arch Surg 112:1003, 1977.

Chinn DH, Filly RA, Callen PW: Congenital diaphragmatic hernia diagnosed prenatally by ultrasound. Radiology 148:119, 1983.

Eraklis AJ, Griscom NT, McGovern JB: Bronchogenic cysts of the mediastinum in infancy. N Engl J Med 281:1150, 1969.

Felker RE, Cartier MS, Emerson DS, et al.: Ultrasound of the fetal thymus. J Ultrasound Med 8:669, 1989.

Massad M, Haddad F, Slim M, et al.: Spinal cord compression in neuroblastoma. Surg Neurol 23:567, 1985.

Newnham JP, Crues JV, Vinstein AL, et al.: Sonographic diagnosis of thoracic gastroenteric cyst in utero. Prenat Diagn 4:467, 1984.

Rasmussen SL, Hwang WS, Harder J, et al.: Intrapericardial teratoma: Ultrasonic and pathological features. J Ultrasound Med 6:159, 1987.

Rempen A, Feige A, Wünsch P: Prenatal diagnosis of bilateral cystic adenomatoid malformation of the lung. J Clin Ultrasound 15:3, 1987.

Fetal Heart

CARDIOMEGALY

Ebstein's anomaly
Tetralogy of Fallot with absent
  pulmonary valve
Cardiomyopathy

DeVore GR, Siasii B, Platt LD: Fetal echocardiography. VIII: Aortic root dilatation—A marker for tetralogy of Fallot. Am J Obstet Gynecol 159:129, 1988.

Kleinman CS, Donnerstein RL, DeVore GR, et al.: Fetal echocardiography for evaluation of in utero congestive heart failure: A technique for study of nonimmune fetal hydrops. N Engl J Med 306:568, 1982.

Lakier JB, Stanger P, Heymann MA, et al.: Tetralogy of Fallot with absent pulmonary valve. Natural history and hemodynamic considerations. Circulation 50:167, 1974.

OVERRIDING AORTA

Tetralogy of Fallot
Pulmonary atresia with VSD
Truncus arteriosus communis
Double-outlet right ventricle

Allan LD, Crawford CC, Anderson RH, et al.: Echocardiographic and anatomical correlations in fetal congenital heart disease. Br Heart J 52:542, 1984.

Kleinman CS, Donnerstein RL, DeVore GR, et al.: Fetal echocardiography for evaluation of in utero congestive heart failure: A technique for study of nonimmune fetal hydrops. N Engl J Med 306:568, 1982.

Riggs TW, Paul MH: Two-dimensional echocardiographic prospective diagnosis of common truncus arteriosus in infants. Am J Cardiol 50:1380, 1982.

FLUID AROUND HEART

Pericardial effusion
Pleural effusion
Normal hypoechoic rim
Arrhythmias
Structural heart disease with gross
    ascites

West MS, Donaldson JS, Shkolnik A: Pulmonary sequestration: Diagnosis by ultrasound. J Ultrasound Med 8:125, 1989.

HEART TUMORS

Comment

Rhabdomyoma
Teratoma
Fibroma
Myxoma
Hemangioma
Mesothelioma
Thickening of chordae tendineae   Clinically insignificant variant
Aneurysm of foramen ovale

Arciniegas E, Hakimi M, Farooki ZQ, et al.: Primary cardiac tumors in children. J Thorac Cardiovasc Surg 79:582, 1980.

Corno A, de Simone G, Catena G, et al.: Cardiac rhabdomyoma: Surgical treatment in the neonate. J Thorac Cardiovasc Surg 87:725, 1984.

Dennis MA, Appareti K, Manco-Johnson ML, et al.: The echocardiographic diagnosis of multiple fetal cardiac tumors. J Ultrasound Med 4:327, 1985.

Gladden JR, Dreiling RJ, Gollub SB, et al.: Two-dimensional echocardiographic features of multiple right atrial myxomas. Am J Cardiol 52:1364, 1983.

Kleinman CS, Donnerstein RL, DeVore GR, et al.: Fetal echocardiography for evaluation of in utero congestive heart failure. A technique for study of nonimmune fetal hydrops. N Engl J Med 306:568, 1982.

Schechter AG, Fakhry J, Shapiro LR, et al.: In utero thickening of the chordae tendineae: A cause of intracardiac echogenic foci. J Ultrasound Med 6:691, 1987.

Schmaltz AA, Apitz J: Primary heart tumors in infancy and childhood. Report of 4 cases and review of literature.Cardiology 67:12, 1981.

Stanford W, Abu-Yousef M, Smith W: Intracardiac tumor (rhabdomyoma) diagnosed by in utero ultrasound: A case report. J Clin Ultrasound 15:337, 1987.

Stewart PA, Wladimiroff JW: Fetal atrial arrhythmias associated with redundancy/aneurysm of the foramen ovale. J Clin Ultrasound 16:643, 1988.

ECTOPIA CORDIS

Pentology of Cantrell
Isolated ectopia cordis

Haynor DR, Shuman WP, Brewer DK, et al.: Imaging of fetal ectopia cordis. Roles of sonography and computed tomography. J Ultrasound Med 3:25, 1984.

Kanagasuntheram R, Verzin JA: Ectopia cordis in man. Thorax 17:159, 1962.

Mercer LJ, Petres RE, Smeltzer JS: Ultrasonic diagnosis of ectopia cordis. Obstet Gynecol 61:523, 1983.

Seeds JW, Cefalo RC, Lies SC, et al.: Early prenatal sonographic appearance of rare thoraco-abdominal eventration. Prenat Diagn 4:437, 1984.

Todros T, Presbitero P, Montemurro D, et al.: Prenatal diagnosis of ectopia cordis. J Ultrasound Med 3:429, 1984.

Wicks JD, Levine MD, Mettler FA: Intrauterine sonography of thoracic ectopia cordis. AJR 137:619, 1981.

ARRHYTHMIAS

	Comment
Atrial extrasystoles	Beats not arising from sinoatrial node; may be conducted to ventricles or blocked
Ventricular extrasystoles	
Paroxysmal supraventricular tachycardia	Rate: 180 to 300 bpm for atrium—all conducted to ventricle; most common in children
Paroxysmal atrial tachycardia	
Atrial flutter	Atrium: 300 to 460 bpm; ventricle slower
Atrial fibrillation	Atrial rate: 400 bpm; ventricle slower

Alan LD, Anderson RH, Sullivan ID, et al.: Evaluation of fetal arrhythmias by echocardiography. Br Heart J 50:240, 1983.

Gleicher N, Elkayam U: Intrauterine dysrhythmias, in Elkayam U, Gleicher N (eds): Cardiac Problems in Pregnancy: Diagnosis and Management of Maternal and Fetal Disease. New York, Alan R. Liss, 1982, pp 535-564.

Hill LM, Breckle R, Driscoll DJ: Sonographic evaluation of prenatal therapy for fetal supraventricular tachycardia and congestive heart failure: A case report. J Reprod Med 28:671, 1983.

Ho SY, Mortimer G, Anderson RH, et al.: Conduction system defects in three perinatal patients with arrhythmia. Br Heart J 53:158, 1985.

Kleinman CS, Copel JA, Weinstein EM, et al.: In utero diagnosis and treatment of fetal supraventricular tachycardia. Sem Perinatol 9:113, 1985.

Kleinman CS, Donnerstein RL, DeVore GR, et al.: Fetal echocardiography for evaluation of in utero congestive heart failure: A technique for study of nonimmune fetal hydrops. N Engl J Med 306:568, 1982.

SHIFT OF HEART

Asplenia/polysplenia
Diaphragmatic hernia
Mass in chest pushing heart
Situs abnormalities
Pleural fluid displacing heart

Campbell S, Pearce JM: The prenatal diagnosis of fetal structural anomalies by ultrasound. Clin Obstet Gynaecol 10:475, 1983.
Chinn DH, Filly RA, Callen PW: Congenital diaphragmatic hernia diagnosed prenatally by ultrasound. Radiology 148:119, 1983.

DEFECT IN ATRIAL SEPTUM

	Comment
Normal	Septum normally difficult to see; may simulate defect
Sinus venosus defect	Near entrance of sinus venosus defect, associated with anomalous pulmonary venous return (APVR)
Ostium secundum defect	Defect at foramen ovale
Ostium primum defect	Outlet portion
Transposition of the great vessels	Associated with atrioventricular (A-V) canal malformations
Pulmonic stenosis	
Asplenia/polysplenia	

Van Mierop LHS, Gessner IH, Schiebler GL: Asplenia and polysplenia syndrome. Birth Defects 8:36, 1972.

DEFECT IN VENTRICULAR SEPTUM

	Comment
Normal	Artifactual ventricular septal defect (VSD) may have edges that fade
VSD	Sharp edges
Tetralogy of Fallot	
Transposition	
Noonan's syndrome	Short stature; cystic hygroma; renal anomalies

Benacerraf BR, Greene MF, Holmes LB: The prenatal sonographic features of Noonan's syndrome. J Ultrasound Med 8:59, 1989.

ATRIOVENTRICULAR SEPTAL DEFECTS

Asplenia

Van Mierop LHS, Gessner IH, Schiebler GL: Asplenia and polysplenia syndrome. Birth Defects 8:36, 1972.

SINGLE VENTRICLE

Univentricular heart
Large VSD
A-V canal
Tricuspid atresia
Mitral atresia
Simulated by hypoplastic right or left
ventricle

Bisset GS, Hirschfeld SS: The univentricular heart: Combined two-dimensional-pulsed Doppler (duplex) echocardiographic evaluation. Am J Cardiol 51:1149, 1983.
Van Praagh R, Ongley PA, Swan HJC: Anatomic types of single or common ventricle in man: Morphologic and geometric aspects of sixty necropsied cases. Am J Cardiol 13:367, 1964.

LARGE RIGHT ATRIUM

Ebstein's anomaly
Idiopathic giant right atrium
Tricuspid valve dysplasia
Premature closure of foramen ovale
Hydrops
Postdates fetus
Ductal constriction
Maternal indomethacin therapy
Tricuspid regurgitation
Ductal constriction

Allan LD, Crawford DC, Anderson RH, et al.: Echocardiographic and anatomical correlations in fetal congenital heart disease. Br Heart J 52:542, 1984.
Fraser WD, Nimrod C, Nicholson S, et al: Antenatal diagnosis of restriction of the foramen ovale. J Ultrasound Med 8:281, 1989.
Murphrey MD, Johnson JA, Mattioli L, et al.: Giant right atrium secondary to tricuspid valve dysplasia in infancy. J Ultrasound Med 4:353, 1985.
Silverman NH, Golbus MS: Echocardiographic techniques for assessing normal and abnormal fetal cardiac anatomy. J Am Coll Cardiol 5:20S, 1985.

SMALL LEFT VENTRICLE

	Comment
Coarctation of aorta	
Hypoplastic left heart	May not see until third trimester
Aortic stenosis	
Total anomalous pulmonary venous return (TAPVR)	
Tetralogy of Fallot	
Critical left heart outflow obstruction	
Noncompliant left ventricle, any cause	
Endocardial fibroelastosis	May have echoes within chambers
Mitral atresia	May have VSD
Aortic atresia	

Benacerraf BR, Saltzman DH, Sanders SP: Sonographic sign suggesting the prenatal diagnosis of coarctation of the aorta. J Ultrasound Med 8:65, 1989.
Hawker RE, Celermajer JM, Gengos DC, et al.: Common pulmonary vein atresia. Premortem diagnosis in two infants. Circulation 46:368, 1972.
Vincent RN, Menticoglou S, Chanas D, et al.: Prenatal diagnosis of an unusual form of hypoplastic left heart syndrome. J Ultrasound Med 6:261, 1987.

SMALL RIGHT VENTRICLE

Pulmonary atresia with intact septum
Pulmonic stenosis
Asplenia
Tricuspid atresia
Hypoplastic right heart

DeVore GR, Siassi B, Platt LD: Fetal echocardiography: The prenatal diagnosis of tricuspid atresia (Type Ic) during the second trimester of pregnancy. J Clin Ultrasound 15:317, 1987.

ENLARGED RIGHT VENTRICLE

Comment

Premature closure of foramen ovale
Pulmonary atresia with intact
  ventricular septum
Pulmonic valve hypoplasia
Total anomalous pulmonary venous
  return
Dysplastic regurgitant tricuspid valve
Coarctation of aorta
Aortic arch anomalies
Normals after 32 weeks
Pulmonary stenosis   From tricuspid regurgitation

DeLeval M, Bull C, Stark J, et al.: Pulmonary atresia and intact ventricular septum: Surgical management based on a revised classification. Circulation 66:272, 1982.

Fraser WD, Nimrod C, Nicholson S, et al.: Antenatal diagnosis of restriction of the foramen ovale. J Ultrasound Med 8:281, 1989.

Lewis AB, Wells W, Lindesmith GG: Evaluation and surgical treatment of pulmonary atresia and intact ventricular septum in infancy. Circulation 67:1318, 1983.

Persutte WH, Yeasting RA, Lenke RR, et al.: Prenatal ultrasonographic appearance of "agenesis" of the ductus arteriosus and pulmonic valve hypoplasia: A case report and review of the embryogenesis. J Ultrasound Med 9:541, 1990.

ENLARGED LEFT VENTRICLE

Aortic stenosis
Variant of hypoplastic left heart
Large for gestational age
Endocardial fibroelastosis (primary)
Mitral insufficiency
Aortic insufficiency

Hawker RE, Celermajer JM, Gengos DC, et al.: Common pulmonary vein atresia. Premortem diagnosis in two infants. Circulation 46:368, 1972.
Vincent RN, Menticoglou S, Chanas D, et al.: Prenatal diagnosis of an unusual form of hypoplastic left heart syndrome. J Ultrasound Med 6:261, 1987.

THICKENED LEFT VENTRICLE WALL

Comment

Tricuspid atresia
Renal disease
Maternal diabetes mellitus
Aortic stenosis
Obstructive cardiomyopathy
Endocardial fibroelastosis   Echogenic myocardium

DeVore GR, Siassi B, Platt LD: Fetal echocardiography: The prenatal diagnosis of tricuspid atresia (Type Ic) during the second trimester of pregnancy. J Clin Ultrasound 15:317, 1987.

THICKENED RIGHT VENTRICLE WALL

Tetralogy of Fallot
Pulmonary stenosis

Nyberg DA, Emerson DS: Cardiac malformations, in Nyberg DA, Mahony BS, Pretorius DH: *Diagnostic Ultrasound of Fetal Anomalies*. Chicago, Yearbook Publishers, 1990, pp 328-329.

ENLARGED PULMONARY ARTERY

Absent pulmonary valve
Total anomalous pulmonary venous
 return
Coarctation of aorta
Tetralogy of Fallot with absent
 pulmonary valve
Pulmonary stenosis

Persutte WH, Yeasting RA, Lenke RR, et al.: Prenatal ultrasonographic appearance of "agenesis" of the ductus arteriosus and pulmonic valve hypoplasia: A case report and review of the embryogenesis. J Ultrasound Med 9:541, 1990.

SMALL PULMONARY ARTERY

Pulmonic stenosis
Tricuspic atresia
Ebstein's anomaly
Tetralogy of Fallot
Pulmonary atresia

SMALL AORTA

	Comment
Aortic stenosis	Especially supravalvular
Hypoplastic left heart	
Coarctation	

ENLARGED AORTA

Aortic stenosis
Tetralogy of Fallot
Pulmonary atresia with VSD
Truncus arteriosus

SMALL LEFT ATRIUM

Comment

TAPVR
Critical pulmonary stenosis (PS) May have small right ventricle (RV)
         also

Fetal Abdomen

ANTERIOR ABDOMINAL WALL DEFECTS OR MASSES

	Comment
Omphalocele	Midline; frequent hepatic herniation; membrane covers mass; umbilical cord enters hernia; increased incidence of neural tube defects
Gastroschisis	Lateral defect; usually right-sided
Pentology of Cantrell	Omphalocele plus ectopic cordis
Beckwith-Wiedemann syndrome	Omphalocele, visceromegaly, and macroglossia
Body-stalk anomaly	No umbilical cord; fetus attached to placenta
Bladder exstrophy	May not see bladder
Cloacal exstrophy	High mortality; have increased incidence of neural tube defects
Normal rotation of gut from 8 to 12 weeks	
Patent urachus	May give extra-abdominal mass
Ectopia cordis	
Vesico-allantoic cyst	Similar to patent urachus

Abu-Yousef MM, Wray AB, Williamson RA, et al.: Antenatal ultrasound diagnosis of variant of Pentalogy of Cantrell. J Ultrasound Med 6:535, 1987.

Barth RA, Filly RA, Sondheimer FK: Prenatal sonographic findings in bladder exstrophy. J Ultrasound Med 9:359, 1990.

Donnenfeld AE, Mennuti MT, Templeton JM, et al.: Prenatal sonographic diagnosis of a vesico-allantoic abdominal wall defect. J Ultrasound Med 8:43, 1989.

Gosden C, Brock DJH: Prenatal diagnosis of exstrophy of the cloaca. Am J Med Genet 8:95, 1981.

Gravier L: Exstrophy of the cloaca. Am Surg 34:387, 1968.

Hasan S, Hermansen MC: The prenatal diagnosis of ventral abdominal wall defects. Am J Obstet Gynecol 155:842, 1986.

Klingensmith WC, Cioffi-Ragan DT, Harvey DE: Diagnosis of ectopia cordis in the second trimester. J Clin Ultrasound 16:204, 1988.

Koontz WL, Shaw LA, Lavery JP: Antenatal sonographic appearance of Beckwith-Wiedemann syndrome. J Clin Ultrasound 14:57, 1986.

Kushnir O, Izquierdo L, Vigil D, et al.: Early transvaginal sonographic diagnosis of gastroschisis. J Clin Ultrasound 18:194, 1990.

Lockwood CJ, Scioscia AL, Hobbins JC: Congenital absence of the umbilical cord resulting from maldevelopment of embryonic body folding. Am J Obstet Gynecol 155:1049, 1986.

Mann L, Ferguson-Smith MA, Desai M, et al.: Prenatal assessment of anterior abdominal wall defects and their prognosis. Prenat Diagn 4:427, 1984.

Mirk P, Calisti A, Fileni A: Prenatal sonographic diagnosis of bladder exstrophy. J Ultrasound Med 5:291, 1986.

Persutte WH, Lenke RR, Kropp K, et al.: Antenatal diagnosis of fetal patent urachus. J Ultrasound Med 7:399, 1988.

Schmidt W, Yarkoni S, Crelin ES, et al.: Sonographic visualization of physiologic anterior abdominal wall hernia in the first trimester. Obstet Gynecol 69:911, 1987.

Seeds JW, Cefalo RC, Lies SC, et al.: Early prenatal sonographic appearance of rare thoraco-abdominal eventration. Prenat Diagn 4:437, 1984.

Weinstein L, Anderson C: In utero diagnosis of Beckwith-Wiedemann syndrome by ultrasound. Radiology 134:474, 1980.

Wood BP: Cloacal malformations and exstrophy syndromes. Radiology 177:326, 1990.

Youngblood JP, Franklin DW, Stein RT: Omphalocele: Early prenatal diagnosis by ultrasound. J Clin Ultrasound 11:339, 1983.

NONVISUALIZATION OF STOMACH

Comment

Tracheoesophageal fistula   May have polyhydramnios
Esophageal atresia
Otocephaly   90% have a stomach

Cayea PD, Bieber FR, Ross MJ, et al.: Sonographic findings in otocephaly (synotia). J Ultrasound Med 4:377, 1985.

Farrant P: The antenatal diagnosis of oesophageal atresia by ultrasound. Br J Radiol 53:1202, 1980.

Jassani MN, Gauderer MWL, Faranoff AA, et al.: A perinatal approach to the diagnosis and management of gastrointestinal malformations. Obstet Gynecol 59:33, 1982.

Pretorius DH, Drose JA, Dennis MA, et al.: Tracheoesophageal fistula in utero: Twenty-two cases. J Ultrasound Med 6:509, 1987.

Rahmani MR, Zalev AH: Antenatal detection of esophageal atresia with distal tracheoesophageal fistula. J Clin Ultrasound 14:143, 1986.

Zemlyn S: Prenatal detection of esophageal atresia. J Clin Ultrasound 9:453, 1981.

FETAL STOMACH MASS

Comment

Vernix   Normal near end of pregnancy
Blood   Especially after abruptio placenta

Walker JM, Ferguson DD: The sonographic appearance of blood in the fetal stomach and its association with placental abruption. J Ultrasound Med 7:155, 1988.

DOUBLE BUBBLE

	Comment
Duodenal atresia	May not be able to diagnose before 20 weeks
Choledochal cyst	No communication between the two cysts
Normal stomach with prominent incisura	
Congenital duplication of stomach	

Balcar I, Grant D, Miller WA, et al.: Antenatal detection of Down syndrome by sonography. AJR 143:29, 1984.

Bidwell JK, Nelson A: Prenatal ultrasonic diagnosis of congenital duplication of the stomach. J Ultrasound Med 5:589, 1986.

Dewbury KC, Aluwihare APR, Birch SJ, et al.: Prenatal ultrasound demonstration of a choledochal cyst. Br J Radiol 53:906, 1980.

Elrad H, Mayden KL, Ahart S, et al.: Prenatal ultrasound diagnosis of choledochal cyst. J Ultrasound Med 4:553, 1985.

Howell CG, Templeton JM, Weiner S, et al.: Antenatal diagnosis and early surgery for choledochal cyst. J Pediatr Surg 18:387, 1983.

Nelson LH, Clark CE, Fishburne JI, et al.: Value of serial sonography in the in utero detection of duodenal atresia. Obstet Gynecol 59:657, 1982.

DILATED LOOPS OF BOWEL

Common

Normal after 22 weeks
Bowel atresia

Uncommon

Congenital chloride diarrhea
Meconium ileus
Cystic fibrosis

Boldstein RB, Filly RA, Callen PW: Sonographic diagnosis of meconium ileus in utero. J Ultrasound Med 6:663, 1987.

Nyberg DA, Hastrup W, Watts H, et al.: Dilated fetal bowel: A sonographic sign of cystic fibrosis. J Ultrasound Med 6:257, 1987.

Nyberg DA, Mack LA, Patten RM, et al.: Fetal bowel: Normal sonographic findings. J Ultrasound Med 6:3, 1987.

Patel PJ, Kolawole TM, Ba'Aqueel HS, et al.: Antenatal sonographic findings of congenital chloride diarrhea. J Clin Ultrasound 17:115, 1989.

ABDOMINAL CYSTS

Common	Comment
Normal fetal bowel	Colon seen as early as 22 weeks
Bowel obstruction	

Uncommon

Duplication cysts	
Intestinal atresia	Look for peristalsis
Hydronephrosis	
Ovarian cysts	
Mesenteric cysts	
Hirschsprung's disease	
Omental cysts	
Pancreatic cysts	
Polycystic kidney disease (adult type)	
Chronic chloride diarrhea	Mainly in Northern Europeans; polyhydramnios
Meconium peritonitis	After perforation, may form cysts
Urachal cysts	
Volvulus of bowel	
Midgut volvulus	
Prenatal appendiceal abscess	
Sacrococcygeal teratoma	
Umbilical vein varices	Fluid collection at level of liver; Doppler shows flow

Bean WJ, Calonje MA, Aprill CN, et al.: Anal atresia: A prenatal ultrasound diagnosis. J Clin Ultrasound 6:111, 1978.

Bidwell JK, Nelson A: Prenatal ultrasonic diagnosis of congenital duplication of the stomach. J Ultrasound Med 5:589, 1986.

Cloutier MG, Fried AM, Selke AC: Antenatal observation of midgut volvulus by ultrasound. J Clin Ultrasound 11:286, 1983.

Crade M, Gillooly L, Taylor KJW: In utero demonstration of an ovarian cystic mass by ultrasound. J Clin Ultrasound 8:251, 1980.

Effmann EL, Griscom NT, Colodny AH, et al.: Neonatal gastrointestinal masses arising late in gestation. Am J Roentgenol 135:681, 1980.

Groli C, Zucca S, Cesaretti A: Congenital chloridorrhea: Antenatal ultrasonographic appearance. J Clin Ultrasound 14:293, 1986.

Hill LM, Breckle R, Avant RF: Sonographic findings associated with sterile fetal appendiceal abscess. J Ultrasound Med 1:257, 1982.

Hill LM, Kislak S, Belfar HL: The sonographic diagnosis of urachal cysts in utero. J Clin Ultrasound 18:434, 1990.

Jeanty P: Fetal and funicular vascular anomalies: Identification with prenatal US. Radiology 173:367, 1989.

Kirkinen P, Jouppila P: Prenatal ultrasonic findings in congenital chloride diarrhea. Prenat Diagn 4:457, 1984.

Kjoller M, Holm-Nielsen G, Meiland H, et al.: Prenatal obstruction of the ileum diagnosed by ultrasound. Prenat Diagn 5:427, 1985.

Nyberg DA, Mack LA, Patten RM, et al.: Fetal bowel: Normal sonographic findings. J Ultrasound Med 6:3, 1987.

Patel PJ, Kolawole TM, Ba'Aqueel HS, et al.: Antenatal sonographic findings of congenital chloride diarrhea. J Clin Ultrasound 17:115, 1989.

Schwimer SR, Vanley GT, Reinke RT: Prenatal diagnosis of cystic meconium peritonitis. J Clin Ultrasound 12:37, 1984.

Sheth S, Nussbaum AR, Sanders RC, et al.: Prenatal diagnosis of sacrococcygeal teratoma: Sonographic-pathologic correlation. Radiology 169:131, 1988.

Vermesch M, Mayden KL, Confino E, et al.: Prenatal sonographic diagnosis of Hirschsprung's disease. J Ultrasound Med 5:37, 1986.

ABDOMINAL MASS*

	Comment
Normal	
Meconium peritonitis	
Midgut volvulus	
Teratomas	
Fetal gallstones	
Complicated ovarian cyst	
Hemangioma	
Hemangioendothelioma	
Hepatoblastoma	
Neuroblastoma	
Teratoma	
Ovarian dermoid	
Toxoplasmosis	
CMV infection	
Infection	
Malignancy	
Sacrococcygeal teratoma	
Trisomy 21	
Normal small bowel	Reported between 16 and 20 weeks
Meconium ileus	
Subdiaphragmatic pulmonary sequestration	
Mesoblastic nephroma	
Wilms' tumor	
Multicystic kidney	
Hepatic hamartoma	
Hydrometrocolpos	
Ovarian cyst	
Urachal cyst	
Mesenteric cyst	
Enteric duplication	
Duodenal atresia	
Dilated bowel	

*Adapted from Romero et al. (1988).

Apuzzio JJ, Unwin W, Adhate A, et al.: Prenatal diagnosis of renal mesoblastic nephroma. Am J Obstet Gynecol 154:636, 1986.

Cloutier MG, Fried AM, Selke AC: Antenatal observation of midgut volvulus by ultrasound. J Clin Ultrasound 11:286, 1983.

Davies P, Ford WDA, Lequesne GW, et al.: Ultrasonic detection of subdiaphragmatic pulmonary sequestration in utero and postnatal diagnosis by fine-needle aspiration biopsy. J Ultrasound Med 8:47, 1989.

Eliezer S, Ester F, Ehund W, et al.: Fetal splenomegaly, ultrasound diagnosis of cytomegalovirus infection: A case report. J Clin Ultrasound 12:520, 1984.

Fakhry J, Reiser M, Shapiro LR, et al.: Increased echogenicity in the lower fetal abdomen: A common normal variant in the second trimester. J Ultrasound Med 5:489, 1986.

Ferraro EM, Fakhry J, Aruny JE, et al.: Prenatal adrenal neuroblastoma: Case report with review of the literature. J Ultrasound Med 7:275, 1988.

Fleischer AC, Davis RJ, Campbell L: Sonographic detection of a meconium-containing mass in a fetus: A case report. J Clin Ultrasound 11:103, 1983.

Goldstein RB, Filly RA, Callen PW: Sonographic diagnosis of meconium ileus in utero. J Ultrasound Med 6:663, 1987.

Jaffe MH, White SJ, Silver TM: Wilms' tumor: Ultrasonic features, pathologic correlation, and diagnostic pitfalls. Radiology 140:147, 1981.

Lince DM, Pretorius DH, Manco-Johnson ML, et al.: The clinical significance of increased echogenicity in the fetal abdomen. AJR 145:683, 1985.

Manco LG, Nunan FA, Sohnen H, et al.: Fetal small bowel simulating an abdominal mass at sonography. J Clin Ultrasound 14:404, 1986.

Persutte WH: Second trimester hyperechogenicity in the lower abdomen of two fetuses with Trisomy 21: Is there a correlation? J Clin Ultrasound 18:425, 1990.

Preziosi P, Fariello G, Maiorana A, et al.: Antenatal sonographic diagnosis of complicated ovarian cysts. J Clin Ultrasound 14:196, 1986.

Romero R, Pilu G, Jeanty P, Ghidini A, Hobbins J: *Prenatal Diagnosis of Congenital Anomalies.* Norwalk, Conn, Appleton & Lange, 1988, pp 244, 299.

Sheth S, Nussbaum AR, Sanders RC, et al.: Prenatal diagnosis of sacrococcygeal teratoma: Sonographic-pathologic correlation. Radiology 169:131, 1988.

Yankes JR, Bowie JD, Effmann EL, et al.: Antenatal diagnosis of meconium peritonitis with inguinal hernias by ultrasonography: Therapeutic implications. J Ultrasound Med 7:221, 1988.

Fetal Liver

HEPATOMEGALY

Common

Hepatitis
CMV infection
Rubella
Congenital hemolytic anemias, such as
   spherocytosis
Isoimmunization
CHF

Uncommon

Toxoplasmosis
Syphilis
Varicella
Coxsackievirus infection
Mesenchymal hamartoma
Hemangioma
Metastatic neuroblastoma
Hepatoblastoma
Hemangiopericytoma
Galactosemia
Tyrosinemia
Alpha-1-antitrypsin deficiency
Disorders of the urea cycle
Methylmalonic acidemia
Infantile sialodosis
Beckwith-Wiedemann syndrome
Zellweger syndrome
Adult polycystic disease of liver and
   kidneys
Solitary cyst

Chung WM: Antenatal detection of hepatic cyst. J Clin Ultrasound 14:217, 1986.
Koontz WL, Shaw LA, Lavery JP: Antenatal sonographic appearance of Beckwith-Wiedemann syndrome. J Clin Ultrasound 14:57, 1986.
Romero R, Pilu G, Jeanty P, Ghidini A, Hobbins J: *Prenatal Diagnosis of Congenital Anomalies.* Norwalk, Conn, Appleton & Lange, 1988, p 250.

Fetal Spleen

SPLENOMEGALY

Common

Viral infection
  CMV
  Rubella
Isoimmunization
Anemia
CHF

Comment

Especially hemolytic

Uncommon

Bacterial infection
Syphilis
Toxoplasmosis
Hepatitis
Leukemia
Lymphoma
Hamartoma
Splenic cysts
Beckwith-Wiedemann syndrome
Gaucher's disease
Niemann-Pick disease
Wolman's disease
Congenital histiocytosis

Eliezer S, Ester F, Ehund W, et al.: Fetal splenomegaly, ultrasound diagnosis of cytomegalovirus infection: A case report. J Clin Ultrasound 12:520, 1984.

Green M: *Pediatric Diagnosis*. Philadelphia, WB Saunders, 1986, pp 92-93.

Koontz WL, Shaw LA, Lavery JP: Antenatal sonographic appearance of Beckwith-Wiedemann syndrome. J Clin Ultrasound 14:57, 1986.

Schmidt W, Yarkoni S, Jeanty P, et al.: Sonographic measurements of the fetal spleen: Clinical implications. J Ultrasound Med 4:667, 1985.

SMALL OR HYPOPLASTIC SPLEEN

Sickle cell disease
DiGeorge's syndrome

Schmidt W, Yarkoni S, Jeanty P, et al.: Sonographic measurements of the fetal spleen: Clinical implications. J Ultrasound Med 4:667, 1985.

Fetal Ascites (by Etiology)*

HEMATOLOGIC

Anemia due to maternal acquired pure
  red cell aplasia
Anemia due to blood loss
  Fetomaternal bleeding
  Twin-to-twin transfusion
Hemolysis: Glucose-6-phosphate
  dehydrogenase deficiency
Hemoglobinopathy: Homozygous
  alpha-thalassemia

PULMONARY

Congenital cystic adenomatoid
  malformation (CCAM)
Pulmonary lymphangiectasia
Pulmonary leiomyosarcoma
Alveolar cell adenoma of the lung
Diaphragmatic hernia
Extralobar pulmonary sequestration
Enlargement of one lung
Chylothorax

NEUROLOGIC

Fetal intracranial hemorrhage
Encephalocele
Porencephaly with absent corpus
  callosum

*Adapted from Romero et al. (1988).

GASTROINTESTINAL

Midgut volvulus
Diaphragmatic hernia
Atresia
  Esophageal with imperforate anus
  Duodenal
  Bowel
  Ileal with meconium peritonitis
Meconium peritonitis with gut
  herniated into peritoneal sac
Meconium peritonitis of unknown
  etiology
Duodenal diverticulum
Imperforate anus

HEPATIC

Cirrhosis with portal hypertension
Giant cell hepatitis
Hepatic necrosis
Hemangioendothelioma of the liver

GENITOURINARY

Congenital nephrotic syndrome
  (Finnish type)
Pelvic kidney
Hypoplastic kidney (with
  microcephaly)
Urethral obstruction with renal
  dysplasia
Hypoplastic uterus, imperforate
  hymen, and bilateral accessory renal
  arteries
Polycystic kidneys, vaginal atresia,
  and hydrocolpos
Urogenital sinus, hydronephrosis, bifid
  uterus, and hydrocolpos
APKD

INFECTIOUS

Coxsackievirus pancarditis
Secondary syphilis
Toxoplasmosis
CMV hepatitis, myocarditis, or
    encephalitis
Parvovirus
Herpes simplex type I
Respiratory syncytial virus
Meconium peritonitis

NEOPLASTIC

Neuroblastoma
Teratoma
Sacral
Mediastinal
Malignant
Congenital leukemia with Down
    syndrome
Hemangioendothelioma of the liver
Pulmonary leiomyosarcoma
Tuberous sclerosis

CARDIOVASCULAR

Cardiac structure
  A-V canal defect
    With abdominal situs inversus and
      complete heart block
    With transposition of great
      arteries
    With transposition of the great
      vessels and asplenia
    With transposition of the great
      vessels and polysplenia
    With double outlet right ventricle
      and pulmonic stenosis
    With overriding aorta and
      tracheoesophageal fistula
    With complex bradyarrhythmia,
      A-V valve insufficiency, and
      interrupted inferior vena cava
      (IVC)
    Complete communication with
      common A-V valve
  Tetralogy of Fallot
  Absent pulmonary valve or
    pulmonary atresia
  Aortic atresia and diminutive left
    ventricle and mitral valve
  Aortic valve stenosis with mitral
    insufficiency
  Aortic arch interruption
  Tricuspid dysplasia and Ebstein's
    anomaly
  Tricuspid and pulmonary atresia
  Myocardial infarction with coronary
    artery embolus
  Intrapericardial teratoma
  Cardiac rhabdomyoma
  Myocardial tumors involving
    ventricular septum, aortic outflow,
    and left atrium, not requiring
    surgery
  Intrauterine closure of foramen
    ovale
  Intrauterine closure of ductus
    arteriosus
Endocardial fibroelastosis
  With mitral valve insufficiency
  With subaortic stenosis

CARDIOVASCULAR (Continued)

Ventricular septal defect (VSD)
  With atrial septal defect (ASD)
  With ASD and right atrial
    conduction system hamartoma
  With patent ductus arteriosus
  With absent right hemidiaphragm
Cardiac rhythm
  Atrial
    Bradycardia and bradyarrhythmia
  Tachycardia
    Paroxysmal (PAT)
    Wolff-Parkinson-White (WPW)
  Flutter with block
Complete heart block
Vascular
  Vena cava thrombosis
  Hemangioendothelioma
  Arterial calcification
  Arteriovenous malformation
  Cerebral angioma

METABOLIC

Gaucher's disease
Sialodosis
Gangliosidosis GM_1
Mucopolysaccharidosis

SKELETAL

Dysplasias
  Achondroplasia
  Achondrogenesis
    Parenti-Fraccaro (or type I)
    Langer-Saldino (or type II)
    Osteogenesis imperfecta
    Thanatophoric dwarfism
    Short rib-polydactyly syndrome
      Saldino-Noonan type
      Majewski type
    Asphyxiating thoracic dysplasia
  Chromosomal
    Triploidy

TRISOMIES

13
21 (Down syndrome)
E
18 (Edwards's syndrome)
Translocation E
47XY + der, t(11:21)(q23:q11)mat
Abnormal chromosome 11
Mosaic 46XX/XY
Mosaic 46XY/92XXYY
45XO (Turner's syndrome)
dup(11p)

HEREDITARY

Pena-Shokeir type I
Lethal multiple pterygium syndrome
Idiopathic
Noonan's syndrome with congenital
heart defect

PLACENTAL

Chorioangioma

Adzick NS, Harrison MR, Flake AW, et al.: Urinary extravasation in the fetus with obstructive uropathy. J Pediatr Surg 20:608, 1985.

Garb M, Rad FF, Riseborough J: Meconium peritonitis presenting as fetal ascites on ultrasound. Br J Radiol 53:602, 1980.

Glazer GM, Filly RA, Callen PW: The varied sonographic appearance of the urinary tract in the fetus and newborn with urethral obstruction. Radiology 144:563, 1982.

Griscom NT, Colodny AH, Rosenberg HK, et al.: Diagnostic aspects of neonatal ascites: Report of 27 cases. AJR 128:961, 1977.

Lubinsky M, Rapoport P: Transient fetal hydrops and "prune belly" in one identical female twin. N Engl J Med 308:256, 1983.

Romero R, Pilu G, Jeanty P, Ghidini A, Hobbins J: *Prenatal Diagnosis of Congenital Anomalies.* Norwalk, Conn, Appleton & Lange, 1988, pp 417-418.

Shapiro I, Sharf M: Spontaneous intrauterine remission of hydrops fetalis in one identical twin: Sonographic diagnosis. J Clin Ultrasound 12:427, 1985.

Vincent RN, Menticoglou S, Chanas D, et al.: Prenatal diagnosis of an unusual form of hypoplastic left heart syndrome. J Ultrasound Med 6:261, 1987.

Fetal Adrenals

MASSES

Adrenal neuroblastoma
Adrenal hemorrhage

Ferraro EM, Fakhry J, Aruny JE, et al.: Prenatal adrenal neuroblastoma: Case report with review of the literature. J Ultrasound Med 7:275, 1988.

Giulian BB, Chang CCN, Yoss BS: Prenatal ultrasonographic diagnosis of fetal adrenal neuroblastoma. J Clin Ultrasound 14:225, 1986.

Fetal Kidneys

ENLARGED KIDNEYS

Common

Infantile polycystic kidney disease
  (IPKD)
Obstruction of kidneys

Uncommon

APKD
Multicystic dysplastic kidneys
Prune-belly syndrome
Beckwith-Wiedemann syndrome
Nephroblastomatosis

Comment

Wilms' tumor precursor

Ambrosino MA, Hernanz-Schulman M, Horii SC, et al.: Prenatal diagnosis of nephroblastomatosis in two siblings. J Ultrasound Med 9:49, 1990.

Bateman BG, Brenbridge ANAG, Buschi AJ: In utero diagnosis of multicystic kidney disease by sonography. J Reprod Med 25:256, 1980.

Beretsky I, Lankin DH, Rusoff JH: Sonographic differentiation between the multicystic dysplastic kidney and the ureteropelvic junction obstruction in utero using high resolution real-time scanners employing digital detection. J Clin Ultrasound 12:429, 1984.

D'Alton M, Romero R, Grannum P, et al.: Antenatal diagnosis of renal anomalies with ultrasound. IV. Bilateral multicystic kidney disease. Am J Obstet Gynecol 54:532, 1986.

Fitzsimons RB, Keohane C, Galvin J: Prune-belly syndrome with ultrasound demonstration of reduction of megacystis in utero. Br J Radiol 58:374, 1985.

Koontz WL, Shaw LA, Lavery JP: Antenatal sonographic appearance of Beckwith-Wiedemann syndrome. J Clin Ultrasound 14:57, 1986.

Meizner I, Bar-Ziv J, Katz M: Prenatal ultrasonic diagnosis of the extreme form of prune-belly syndrome. J Clin Ultrasound 13:581, 1985.

Romero R, Cullen M, Jeanty P, et al.: The diagnosis of congenital renal anomalies with ultrasound. II. Infantile polycystic kidney disease. Am J Obstet Gynecol 150:259, 1984.

Shih WJ, Greenbaum LD, Baro C: In utero sonogram in prune-belly syndrome. Urology 20:102, 1982.

Simpson JL, Sabbagha RE, Elias S, et al.: Failure to detect polycystic kidneys in utero by second trimester ultrasonography. Hum Genet 60:295, 1982.

Sumner E, Volberg FM, Martin JF: Real-time sonography of congenital cystic kidney disease. Urology 20:97, 1982.

CYSTS IN KIDNEYS

Obstruction
APKD
Multicystic dysplastic kidneys
Obstruction of kidneys
Prune belly (Eagle Barrett syndrome)
Duplicated system with obstructed
upper pole

Bateman BG, Brenbridge ANAG, Buschi AJ: In utero diagnosis of multicystic kidney disease by sonography. J Reprod Med 25:256, 1980.

Beretsky I, Lankin DH, Rusoff JH: Sonographic differentiation between the multicystic dysplastic kidney and the ureteropelvic junction obstruction in utero using high resolution real-time scanners employing digital detection. J Clin Ultrasound 12:429, 1984.

D'Alton M, Romero R, Grannum P, et al.: Antenatal diagnosis of renal anomalies with ultrasound. IV. Bilateral multicystic kidney disease. Am J Obstet Gynecol 54:532, 1986.

Fitzsimons RB, Keohane C, Galvin J: Prune-belly syndrome with ultrasound demonstration of reduction of megacystis in utero. Br J Radiol 58:374, 1985.

Meizner I, Bar-Ziv J, Katz M: Prenatal ultrasonic diagnosis of the extreme form of prune-belly syndrome. J Clin Ultrasound 13:581, 1985.

Shih WJ, Greenbaum LD, Baro C: In utero sonogram in prune-belly syndrome. Urology 20:102, 1982.

Sherer DM, Menashe M, Lebensart P, et al.: Sonographic diagnosis of unilateral fetal renal duplication with associated ectopic ureterocele. J Clin Ultrasound 17:371, 1989.

ECHOGENIC KIDNEYS

Comment

IPKD
Fetal renal vein thrombosis

Punctate or streaky areas of increased echoes

Lalmand B, Avni EF, Nasr A, et al.: Perinatal renal vein thrombosis: Sonographic demonstration. J Ultrasound Med 9:437, 1990.

Patel RB, Connors JJ: In utero sonographic findings in fetal renal vein thrombosis with calcifications. J Ultrasound Med 7:349, 1988.

HYDRONEPHROSIS

Common	Comment
Normal	Especially after 24 weeks
Uteropelvic junction (UPJ) obstruction	
Uterovesical junction (UVJ) obstruction	
Overdistended fetal bladder	
Posterior urethral valves	
Vesicoureteral reflux	

Uncommon	
Primary megaureter	May have polyhydramnios
Prune-belly syndrome	

Dunn V, Glasier CM: Ultrasonographic antenatal demonstration of primary megaureters. J Ultrasound Med 4:101, 1985.

Hoddick WK, Filly RA, Mahony BS, et al.: Minimal fetal renal pyelectasis. J Ultrasound Med 4:85, 1985.

EMPTY RENAL FOSSA

	Comment
Renal agenesis	Other kidney enlarged
Crossed fused ectopia	Look at other kidney
Pelvic kidneys	

Jeanty P, Romero R, Kepple D, et al.: Prenatal diagnoses in unilateral empty renal fossa. J Ultrasound Med 9:651, 1990.

Fetal Bladder

NONVISUALIZATION OF BLADDER

Common

Bilateral renal agenesis
Polycystic kidney disease

Comment

Severe oligohydramnios

Uncommon

Bladder exstrophy
Multicystic kidneys (bilateral)
Bilateral UPJ obstruction

Normal amount of amniotic fluid
Severe oligohydramnios

Hadlock FP, Deter RL, Carpenter R, et al.: Review. Sonography of fetal urinary tract anomalies. AJR 137:261, 1981.

Keirse MJNC, Meerman RH: Antenatal diagnosis of Potter syndrome. Obstet Gynecol 52:64S, 1978.

Miskin M: Prenatal diagnosis of renal agenesis by ultrasonography and maternal pyelography. AJR 132:1025, 1979.

Romero R, Cullen M, Grannum P, et al.: Antenatal diagnosis of renal anomalies with ultrasound. III. Bilateral renal agenesis. Am J Obstet Gynecol 151:38, 1985.

Romero R, Cullen M, Jeanty P, et al.: The diagnosis of congenital renal anomalies with ultrasound. II. Infantile polycystic kidney disease. Am J Obstet Gynecol 150:259, 1984.

Simpson JL, Sabbagha RE, Elias S, et al.: Failure to detect polycystic kidneys in utero by second trimester ultrasonography. Hum Genet 60:295, 1982.

Sumner E, Volberg FM, Martin JF: Real-time sonography of congenital cystic kidney disease. Urology 20:97, 1982.

DISTENDED BLADDER

Common	*Comment*
Posterior urethral valves	

Uncommon

Megacystic-microcolon-intestinal syndrome	Hypoperistalsis
Absence of urethra	
Caudal regression	

Berdon WE, Baker DH, Blanc WA, et al.: Megacystis-microcolon-intestinal hypoperistalsis syndrome: A new cause of intestinal obstruction in the newborn. Report of radiologic findings in five newborn girls. AJR 126:957, 1976.

Manco LG, Osterdahl P: The antenatal sonographic features of megacystis-microcolon-intestinal hypoperistalsis syndrome. J Clin Ultrasound 12:595, 1984.

Vezina WC, Morin FR, Winsberg F: Megacystis-microcolon-intestinal hypoperistalsis syndrome: Antenatal ultrasound appearance. AJR 133:749, 1979.

Vintzileos AM, Eisenfeld LI, Herson VC, et al.: Megacystis-microcolon-intestinal hypoperistalsis syndrome—Prenatal sonographic findings and review of the literature. Am J Perinatol 3:297, 1986.

Young LW, Yunis EJ, Girdany BR, et al.: Megacystis-microcolon-intestinal hypoperistalsis syndrome: Additional clinical radiologic, surgical, and histopathologic aspects. AJR 137:749, 1981.

Fetal Pelvis

MASSES

Common	Comment
Hydrometrocolpos	Cystic or complex
Ovarian cyst	
Dilated bowel	
Myelomeningocele	

Uncommon

Ovarian tumor	
Chordoma	
Distended rectum	
Urachal cyst	Anterior; midline
Mesenteric cyst	
Enteric duplication	
Sacrococcygeal teratoma	May be cystic, solid, or mixed; one third are calcified
Wolffian duct cyst	
Bowel perforation	
Ovarian torsion	

Crade M, Gillooly L, Taylor KJM: In utero demonstration of an ovarian cyst mass by ultrasound. J Clin Ultrasound 8:251, 1980.

Davis GH, Wapner RJ, Kurtz AB, et al.: Antenatal diagnosis of hydrometrocolpos by ultrasound examination. J Ultrasound Med 3:371, 1984.

Ein SH, Adeyemi SD, Mancer K: Benign sacrococcygeal teratomas in infants and children. A 25-year review. Ann Surg 191:382, 1980.

Hill SJ, Hirsch JH: Sonographic detection of fetal hydrometrocolpos. J Ultrasound Med 4:323, 1985.

Hogge WA, Thiagarajah S, Barber VG, et al.: Cystic sacrococcygeal teratoma: Ultrasound diagnosis and perinatal management. J Ultrasound Med 6:707, 1987.

Holzgreve W, Mahony BS, Glick PL, et al.: Sonographic demonstration of fetal sacrococcygeal teratoma. Prenat Diagn 5:245, 1985.

Kapoor R, Saha MM, Mandal AK: Antenatal sonographic detection of Wolffian duct cyst. J Clin Ultrasound 17:515, 1989.

Lees RF, Williamson BR, Brenbridge NA, et al.: Sonography of benign sacral teratoma in utero. Radiology 134:717, 1980.

Lockwood C, Ghindini A, Romero R, et al.: Fetal bowel perforation simulating sacrococcygeal teratoma. J Ultrasound Med 7:227, 1988.

Nussbaum AR, Sanders RC, Hartman DS, et al.: Neonatal ovarian cysts: Sonographic-pathologic correlation. Radiology 168:817, 1988.

Preziosi P, Fariello G, Maiorana A, et al.: Antenatal sonographic diagnosis of complicated ovarian cysts. J Clin Ultrasound 14:196, 1986.

Russ PD, Zavitz WR, Pretorius DH, et al.: Hydrometrocolpos, uterus didelphys, and septate vagina: An antenatal sonographic diagnosis. J Ultrasound Med 5:211, 1986.

Sandler MA, Smith SJ, Pope SG, et al.: Prenatal diagnosis of septated ovarian cysts. J Clin Ultrasound 13:55, 1985.

Seeds JW, Mittelstaedt A, Cefalo RC, et al.: Prenatal diagnosis of sacrococcygeal teratoma: An anechoic caudal mass. J Clin Ultrasound 10:193, 1982.

Sherer DM, Shah YG, Eggers PC, et al.: Prenatal sonographic diagnosis and subsequent management of fetal adnexal torsion. J Ultrasound Med 9:161, 1990.

Valdiserri RO, Yunis EJ: Sacrococcygeal teratomas: A review of 68 cases. Cancer 48:217, 1981.

Fetal Skeleton

SKELETAL DYSPLASIAS

	Comment
Extreme micromelia	
Achondrogenesis	
Thanatophoric dysplasia	Telephone receiver femur
Fibrochondrogenesis	
Atelosteogenesis	
Short rib-polydactyly syndromes	
Diastrophic dysplasia	
Dyssegmental dysplasia	
Robert's syndrome	
Hypophosphatasia	Decreased ossification also
Rhizomelia	
Thanatophoric dysplasia	Telephone receiver femur
Atelosteogenesis	
Chondrodysplasia punctate rhizometic type	
Diastrophic dysplasia	
Congenital short femur	
Mesomelia	
Mesomelic dysplasia	Also known as Robinow's syndrome
Acromesomelia	
Ellis-van Creveld syndrome	
Metaphyseal flaring (dumbbell-shaped bones)	
Metatropic dysplasia	
Kneist syndrome	
Dyssegmental dysplasia	
Weissenbacher-Zweymuller syndrome	
Fibrochondrogenesis	
Short rib-polydactyly syndrome type III	
Curved or bowed long bones	
Normal physiologic bowing	
Camptomelic syndrome	
Osteogenesis imperfecta	
Dyssegmental dysplasia	
Otopalatodigital syndrome	
Thanatophoric dysplasia	Telephone receiver femur

Robert's syndrome
Hypophosphatasia
Bone fractures
  Osteogenesis imperfecta
  Hypophosphatasia
  Achondrogenesis
Hypoplastic or absent fibula
  Fibrochondrogenesis
  Atelosteogenesis
  Mesomelic dysplasia: Langer's and
    Reinhart's types
  Otopalatodigital syndrome
Hypoplastic scapulae
  Camptomelic syndrome
Normal long bones
  Larsen's syndrome
  Cleidocranial dysplasia
  Craniosynostoses
  Arthrogryposis multiplex congenita
  Jarcho-Levin syndrome
Clubfoot deformity
  Diastrophic dysplasia
  Osteogenesis imperfecta
  Kneist dysplasia
  Spondyloepiphysial congenita
  Metatropic dysplasia
  Mesomelic dysplasia, Neivergeit
    type
  Chondrodysplasia punctate
  Robert's syndrome
  Pena-Shokeir syndrome

Polyhydramnios, IUGR, ankyloses,
  and pulmonary hypoplasia

  Arthrogryposis multiplex congenita
  Larsen's syndrome
Postaxial polydactyly
  Chondroectodermal dysplasia
  Short rib-polydactyly syndromes
Preaxial polydactyly
  Chondroectodermal dysplasia
  Short rib-polydactyly syndromes
Hitchhiker thumbs
  Diastrophic dysplasia
Long, narrow thorax
  Asphyxiating thoracic dysplasia
  Chondroectodermal dysplasia
  Metatropic dysplasia
  Fibrochondrogenesis
  Atelosteogenesis

SKELETAL DYSPLASIAS (Continued)

    Camptomelic dysplasia
    Achondrogenesis
    Hypophosphatasia
    Cleidocranial dysplasia
Hypoplastic thorax
    Short rib-polydactyly syndromes
    Thanatophoric dysplasia
    Homozygous achondroplasia

DeLange M, Rouse GA: Prenatal diagnosis of hypophosphatasia. J Ultrasound Med 9:115, 1990.
Genkins SM, Hertzberg BS, Bowie JD, et al.: Pena-Shokeir Type I syndrome: In utero sonographic appearance. J Clin Ultrasound 17:56, 1989.
Graham D, Tracey J, Winn K, et al.: Early second trimester sonographic diagnosis of achondrogenesis. J Clin Ultrasound 11:336, 1983.
Skiptunas SM, Weiner S: Early prenatal diagnosis of asphyxiating thoracic dysplasia (Jeune's syndrome). J Ultrasound Med 6:41, 1987.

DECREASED OSSIFICATION, CALVARIUM

Achondrogenesis
Hypophosphatasia

Romero R, Pilu G, Jeanty P, Ghidini A, Hobbins J: *Prenatal Diagnosis of Congenital Anomalies.* Norwalk, Conn, Appleton & Lange, 1988, pp 357-358.

MULTIPLE CONTRACTURES

                                    Comment

Diastrophic dysplasia	
Arthrogryposis multiplex congenita	Due to lack of movement
Mesomelic dysplasia, Neivergeit type	
Pena-Shokeir I	Ankyloses, clubfeet, camptodactyly, pulmonary hypoplasia, IUGR, and polyhydramnios

Genkins SM, Hertzberg BS, Bowie JD, et al.: Pena-Shokeir Type I syndrome: In utero sonographic appearance. J Clin Ultrasound 17:56, 1989.

CLUBFOOT*

Common	Comment
Amyoplasia congenita disruptive sequence	
Diastrophic dysplasia syndrome	
Distal arthrogryposis syndrome	
Escobar syndrome	Webbing; short stature; oral-facial anomalies
Femoral hypoplasia	Unusual facies syndrome
Fetal aminopterin effects	Varus; cranial-facial dysmorphism; short stature; spina bifida
Freeman-Sheldon syndrome	Varus with contracted toes; multiple skeletal anomalies
Hecht syndrome	
Larsen's syndrome	Hypertelorism; joint laxity; cleft palate; congenital heart disease
Meckel-Gruber syndrome	Microcephaly; cleft palate; encephalocele
Moebius sequence	Limb anomalies
Partial trisomy 10q syndrome	
Pena-Shokeir I syndrome	Hydrops; small chest; short long bones; flexion deformities
Triploidy syndrome	
Trisomy 9 mosaic syndrome	
Trisomy 9p syndrome	
Trisomy 20p syndrome	
Zellweger syndrome	Bell-shaped thorax; limb anomalies
4p − syndrome	Microcephaly; hypertelorism
9p − syndrome	
13q − syndrome	
18q − syndrome	

Uncommon

Aarskog's syndrome	Maxillary hypoplasia
Bloom's syndrome	
Conradi-Hünermann syndrome	Short long bones; fetal ascites
Dubowitz syndrome	
Ehlers-Danlos syndrome	
Ellis-van Creveld syndrome	Valgus; polydactyly; short ribs
Generalized gangliosidosis syndrome	
Homocystinuria syndrome	Pes cavus; everted feet; microcephaly
Hunter's syndrome	

*Adapted from Romero et al. (1988).

CLUBFOOT (Continued)

Uncommon	*Comment*
Mietens syndrome	Skeletal anomalies
Nail-patella syndrome	GU anomalies
Noonan's syndrome	Short stature; cardiovascular anomalies; web neck
Radial aplasia–thrombocytopenia syndrome	
Riley-Day syndrome	
Schwartz syndrome	
Seckel's syndrome	Microcrania
Steinert myotonic dystrophy syndrome	
Trisomy 4p syndrome	
Trisomy 13 syndrome	
Trisomy 18 syndrome	
Weaver syndrome	
XXXXX syndrome	
XXXXY syndrome	
18 − syndrome	
Amniotic band syndrome	

Romero R, Pilu G, Jeanty P, Ghidini A, Hobbins J: *Prenatal Diagnosis of Congenital Anomalies.* Norwalk, Conn, Appleton & Lange, 1988, pp 131, 377.

WIDENED METAPHYSES

	Comment
Metatrophic dysplasia	Flared or dumbbell-shaped bones
Weisenbacher-Zweymuller syndrome	Micromelia, micrognathia, and cleft in vertebrae
Fibrochondrogenesis	
Kneist syndrome	
Dyssegmental dysplasia	

Crowle P, Astley R, Insley J: A form of metatropic dwarfism in two brothers. Pediatr Radiol 4:172, 1976.

Dinno ND, Shearer L, Weisskopf B: Chondrodysplastic dwarfism, cleft palate and micrognathia in a neonate. A new syndrome? Eur J Pediatr 123:39, 1976.

Gruhn JG, Gorlin RJ, Langer LO Jr: Dyssegmental dwarfism. A lethal anisospondylic camptomicromelic dwarfism. Am J Dis Child 132:382, 1978.

Langer LO Jr, Gonzalez-Ramos M, Chen H, et al.: A severe infantile micromelic chondrodysplasia which resembles Kneist disease. Eur J Pediatr 123:29, 1976.

Rimoin DL, Siggers DC, Lachman RS, Silberberg R: Metatropic dwarfism, the Kneist syndrome and the pseudoachondroplastic dysplasias. Clin Orthop 114:70, 1976.

BONE DEMINERALIZATION

Comment

Osteogenesis imperfecta
Hypophosphatasia

Especially in vertebral bodies

Aylsworth AS, Seeds JW, Bonner-Guilford W, et al.: Prenatal diagnosis of a severe deforming type of osteogenesis imperfecta. Am J Med Genet 19:707, 1984.

Chervenak FA, Romero R, Berkowitz RL, et al.: Antenatal sonographic findings of osteogenesis imperfecta. Am J Obstet Gynecol 143:228, 1982.

DeLange M, Rouse GA: Prenatal diagnosis of hypophosphatasia. J Ultrasound Med 9:115, 1990.

Elejalde BR, de Elejalde MM: Prenatal diagnosis of perinatally lethal osteogenesis imperfecta. Am J Med Genet 14:353, 1983.

Ghosh A, Woo JSK, Wan CW, et al.: Simple ultrasonic diagnosis of osteogenesis imperfecta type II in early second trimester. Prenat Diagn 4:235, 1984.

Hobbins JC, Bracken MB, Mahoney MJ: Diagnosis of fetal skeletal dysplasias with ultrasound. Am J Obstet Gynecol 142:306, 1982.

Mertz E, Goldhofer W: Sonographic diagnosis of lethal osteogenesis imperfecta in the second trimester: Case report and review. J Clin Ultrasound 14:380, 1986.

Robinson LP, Worthen NJ, Lachman RS, et al.: Prenatal diagnosis of osteogenesis imperfecta type III. Prenat Diagn 7:7, 1987.

Spranger J, Cremin B, Beighton P: Osteogenesis imperfecta congenita. Features and prognosis of a heterogeneous condition. Pediatr Radiol 12:21, 1982.

JOINT LAXITY/DISLOCATION

Larsen's syndrome

Habermann ET, Sterling A, Dennis RI: Larsen syndrome: A heritable disorder. J Bone Joint Surg 58:558, 1976.

Maroteaux P: Heterogeneity of Larsen's syndrome. Arch Fr Pediatr 32:597, 1975.

Micheli LJ, Hall JE, Watts HG: Spinal instability in Larsen's syndrome: Report of three cases. J Bone Joint Surg 58:526, 1976.

Oki T, Terashima Y, Murachi S, et al.: Clinical features and treatment of joint dislocations in Larsen's syndrome. Report of three cases in one family. Clin Orthop 119:206, 1976.

POLYDACTYLY

Common	Comment
Carpenter's syndrome	
Ellis-van Creveld syndrome	Short ribs
Meckel-Gruber syndrome	Microcephaly; cleft palate; encephalocele
Polysyndactyly syndrome	
Towne syndrome	
Trisomy 13 syndrome	
Short rib-polydactyly syndrome	Short ribs and small thorax

Uncommon

Bloom's syndrome	
Conradi-Hünermann syndrome	Short long bones; fetal ascites
Goltz syndrome	Microcephaly; rib anomalies; renal anomalies
Klippel-Trenaunay-Weber syndrome	Long limb; soft-tissue prominence
Oral-facial-digital syndrome	
Partial trisomy 10q syndrome	
Rubinstein-Taybi syndrome	
Smith-Lemli-Opitz syndrome	
Trisomy 4p syndrome	
Cleft lip-cleft palate	
Asphyxiating thoracic dystrophy	
Congenital mesoblastic nephroma	
McKusick-Kaufman syndrome	Hydrometrocolpos, polydactyly, and heart defects
Lissencephaly	
Werner syndrome	No thumbs; hypoplastic tibia
Otopalatodigital syndrome	Cleft palate, bowed long bones; associated with single umbilical artery

Brewster TG, Lachman RS, Kushner DC, et al.: Otopalato-digital syndrome, Type II — An X-linked skeletal dysplasia. Am J Med Genet 20:249, 1985.

Chervenak FA, Tortora M, Mayden K, et al.: Antenatal diagnosis of median cleft face syndrome: Sonographic demonstration of cleft lip and hypertelorism. Am J Obstet Gynecol 149:94, 1984.

Howell CG, Othersen HB, Kiviat NE, et al.: Therapy and outcome in 51 children with mesoblastic nephroma: A report of the national Wilms' tumor study. J Pediatr Surg 17:826, 1982.

Meholic AJ, Freimanist KA, Stucka J, Lo Piccolo ML: Sonographic in utero diagnosis of Klippel-Trenaunay-Weber syndrome. J Ultrasound Med 10:111, 1991.

Opitz JM: Lissencephaly syndrome, in Bergsma D (ed): Birth Defects Compendium, 2d ed. New York, Alan R Liss, 1979, p 658.

Pashayan H, Fraser FC, McIntyre JM, et al.: Bilateral aplasia of the tibia, polydactyly and absent thumbs in father and daughter. J Bone Joint Surg 53B:495, 1971.

Robinow M, Shaw A: The McKusick-Kaufman syndrome: Recessively inherited vaginal atresia, hydrometrocolpos, uterovaginal duplications, anorectal anomalies, postaxial polydactyly and congenital heart disease. J Pediatr 94:776, 1979.

Romero R, Pilu G, Jeanty P, Ghidini A, Hobbins J: *Prenatal Diagnosis of Congenital Anomalies.* Norwalk, Conn, Appleton & Lange, 1988, p 376.

Schinzel A, Savoldelli G, Briner J, et al.: Prenatal sonographic diagnosis of Jeune syndrome. Radiology 154:777, 1985.

CLAVICULAR HYPOPLASIA

	Comment
Sprengel's deformity, Klippel-Feil syndrome	Minimal; inconsistent; rare hypoplasia
Skeletal dysostosis	Significant hypoplasia or agenesis
Chromosome disorder (11q partial trisomy, 11q/22q partial trisomy, 20p trisomy)	
Multiple congenital anomalies	
Dysplasia cleidofacialis	
Digit-mandible-clavicle hypoplasia	
Microcephaly-micrognathia-contracture dwarfism	
Imperforate anus-psoriasis-clavicle deficiency	
Robert's syndrome, Holt-Oram syndrome, thrombocytopenia–radial aplasia	Associated with significant upper limb deficiency
Achondrogenesis, hyperplastic osteogenesis imperfecta, others	Associated with lethal neonatal dwarfism

Romero R, Pilu G, Jeanty P, Ghidini A, Hobbins J: *Prenatal Diagnosis of Congenital Anomalies.* Norwalk, Conn, Appleton & Lange, 1988, p 368.

ABSENCE OF LIMB OR SEGMENT OF LIMB

Robert's syndrome
Holt-Oram syndrome
Thrombocytopenia
Amniotic band syndrome
Reduction deformity of four limbs
Hypoplastic radius
Absent radii bilateral

Romero R, Pilu G, Jeanty P, Ghidini A, Hobbins J: *Prenatal Diagnosis of Congenital Anomalies.* Norwalk, Conn, Appleton & Lange, 1988, pp 374-376, 414.

ENLARGED LIMB

Hemangioma
Lymphangioma
Klippel-Trenaunay-Weber syndrome
Soft tissue sarcomas

Suma V, Marini A, Gamba PG, et al.: Giant hemangioma of the thigh: Prenatal sonographic diagnosis. J Clin Ultrasound 18:421, 1990.
Warhit JM, Goldman MA, Sachs L, et al.: Klippel-Trenaunay-Weber syndrome: Appearance in utero. J Ultrasound Med 2:515, 1983.

ROCKER-BOTTOM FEET

Comment

Trisomy 18
18q− syndrome
Cerebrooculofacioskeletal syndrome   Large head; plantar surface convex

---

Romero R, Pilu G, Jeanty P, Ghidini A, Hobbins J: *Prenatal Diagnosis of Congenital Anomalies.* Norwalk, Conn, Appleton & Lange, 1988, p 379.

Fluid Abnormalities*

POLYHYDRAMNIOS

Common

Idiopathic
Neural tube defects
Twin pregnancy

Uncommon

	Comment
Chylothorax	
Lung sequestration	
Diaphragmatic hernia	
Beckwith-Wiedemann syndrome	Enphalocele; organomegaly; macroglossia
Esophageal atresia	
Otocephaly	
Duodenal atresia	
Intestinal atresia	
Meconium peritonitis	
Megacystis-microcolon-hypoperistalsis intestinal syndrome	
Congenital chloride diarrhea	Dilated loops of small and large bowel
Cleft palate	
Congenital mesoblastic nephroma	
Intestinal obstruction	
Ovarian cysts	
Asphyxiating thoracic dysplasia	
Robert's syndrome	
Lissencephaly	
Large bladder obstructing bowel	
Vesico-ureteral reflux	
Tracheo-esophageal fistula	Absent stomach
Fetal goiter	
Fetal neck mass	
Neck teratoma	
Chorioangioma of placenta	
Noonan's syndrome	Cystic hygromas; renal and cardiac anomalies

*Adapted from Romero et al. (1988).

165

Anderson EA, Hertel J, Pedersen SA, et al.: Congenital chylothorax: Management by ligature of the thoracic duct. Scand J Thorac Cardiovas Surg 18:193, 1984.

Barone CM, Van Natta FC, Kourides IA, et al.: Sonographic detection of fetal goiter, an unusual cause of hydramnios. J Ultrasound Med 4:625, 1985.

Barss VA, Benacerraf BR, Frigoletto FD: Second trimester oligohydramnios, a predictor of poor fetal outcome. Obstet Gynecol 64:608, 1984.

Benacerraf BR, Greene MF, Holmes LB: The prenatal sonographic features of Noonan's syndrome. J Ultrasound Med 8:59, 1989.

Biedel CW, Pagon RA, Zapata JO: Mullerian anomalies and renal agenesis: Autosomal dominant urogenital adysplasia. J Pediatr 104:861, 1984.

Biedner B: Potter's syndrome with ocular anomalies. J Pediatr Ophthalmol Strabismus 17:172, 1980.

Blank E, Neerbout RC, Burry KA: Congenital mesoblastic nephroma and polyhydramnios. JAMA 240:1504, 1978.

Buchta RM, Viseskul C, Gilbert EF, et al.: Familial bilateral renal agenesis and hereditary renal adysplasia. Z Kinderheilk 115:111, 1973.

Bundy AL, Saltzman DH, Emerson D, et al.: Sonographic features associated with cleft palate. J Clin Ultrasound 14:486, 1986.

Cayea PD, Bieber FR, Ross MJ, et al.: Sonographic findings in otocephaly (synotia). J Ultrasound Med 4:377, 1985.

Dillard JP, Edwards DK, Leopold GR: Meconium peritonitis masquerading as fetal hydrops. J Ultrasound Med 6:49, 1987.

Duenhoelter JH, Santos-Ramos R, Rosenfeld CR, et al.: Prenatal diagnosis of gastrointestinal tract obstruction. Obstet Gynecol 47:618, 1976.

Farrant P: The antenatal diagnosis of oesophageal atresia by ultrasound. Br J Radiol 53:1202, 1980.

Fleischer AC, Killam AP, Boehm FH, et al.: Hydrops fetalis: Sonographic evaluation and clinical implications. Radiology 141:163, 1981.

Groli C, Zucca S, Cesaretti A: Congenital chloridorrhea: Antenatal ultrasonographic appearance. J Clin Ultrasound 14:293, 1986.

Hurwitz A, Yagel S, Rabinovitz R, et al.: Hydramnios caused by pure megacystis. J Clin Ultrasound 12:110, 1984.

Jassani MN, Gauderer MWL, Faranoff AA, et al.: A perinatal approach to the diagnosis and management of gastrointestinal malformations. Obstet Gynecol 59:33, 1982.

Jouppila P, Kirkinen P, Herva R, et al.: Prenatal diagnosis of pleural effusions by ultrasound. J Clin Ultrasound 11:516, 1984.

Koontz WL, Shaw LA, Lavery JP: Antenatal sonographic appearance of Beckwith-Wiedemann syndrome. J Clin Ultrasound 14:57, 1986.

Optiz JM: Lissencephaly syndrome, in Bergsma D (ed): *Birth Defects Compendium*, 2d ed. New York, Alan R Liss, 1979, p 658.

Patel PJ, Kolawole TM, Ba'Aqueel HS, et al.: Antenatal sonographic findings of congenital chloride diarrhea. J Clin Ultrasound 17:115, 1989.

Philipson EH, Wolfson RN, Kedia KR: Fetal hydronephrosis and polyhydramnios associated with vesico-ureteral reflux. J Clin Ultrasound 12:585, 1984.

Pretorius DH, Drose JA, Dennis MA, et al.: Tracheoesophageal fistula in utero: Twenty-two cases. J Ultrasound Med 6:509, 1987.

Rahmani MR, Zalev AR: Antenatal detection of esophageal atresia with distal tracheoesophageal fistula. J Clin Ultrasound 14:143, 1986.

Rosenfeld CR, Coln CD, Duenhoelter JH: Fetal cervical teratoma as a cause of polyhydramnios. Pediatrics 64:176, 1979.

Smith DW: *Recognizable Patterns of Human Malformation. Genetic, Embryologic and Clinical Aspects.* Philadelphia, WB Saunders, 1982, p 221.

Tabsh KMA: Antenatal sonographic appearance of a fetal ovarian cyst. J Ultrasound Med 1:329, 1982.

Trecet JC, Claramunt V, Larraz J, et al.: Prenatal ultrasound diagnosis of fetal teratoma of the neck. J Clin Ultrasound 12:509, 1984.

Weinstein L, Anderson C: In utero diagnosis of Beckwith-Wiedemann syndrome by ultrasound. Radiology 134:474, 1980.

Wolfe BK, Kirk Wallace JH: Pitfall to avoid: Chorioangioma of the placenta simulating fetal tumor. J Clin Ultrasound 15:405, 1987.

Zemlyn S: Prenatal detection of esophageal atresia. J Clin Ultrasound 9:453, 1981.

OLIGOHYDRAMNIOS

Common

Comment

Bilateral renal agenesis
Polycystic kidney disease (infantile or
  adult)
Renal obstruction
Bladder obstruction
Premature rupture of membranes
Intrauterine growth retardation

Uncommon

Multicystic dysplastic kidney
  (bilateral)
Prune-belly syndrome
Caudal regression
Absence of urethra
Triploidy
Sirenomelia   Mermaid fetus
Triploid fetus

Atwell JD: Posterior urethral valves in the British Isles: A multicenter B.A.P.S. review. J Pediatr Surg
  18:70, 1983.
Bellinger MF, Comstock CH, Grosso D, et al.: Fetal posterior urethral valves and renal dysplasia at 15
  weeks gestational age. J Urol 129:1238, 1983.
Crane JP, Beaver HA, Cheung SW: Antenatal ultrasound findings in fetal triploidy syndrome. J Ultrasound Med 4:519, 1985.
Dean WM, Bourdeau EJ: Amniotic fluid alphafetoprotein in fetal obstructive uropathy. Pediatrics 60:537,
  1980.
Fitzsimons RB, Keohane C, Galvin J: Prune-belly syndrome with ultrasound demonstration of reduction
  of megacystis in utero. Br J Radiol 58:374, 1985.
Glazer GM, Filly RA, Callen PW: The varied sonographic appearance of the urinary tract in the fetus
  and newborn with urethral obstruction. Radiology 144:563, 1982.
Hadlock FP, Deter RL, Carpenter R, et al.: Review. Sonography of fetal urinary tract anomalies. AJR
  137:261, 1981.
Keirse MJNC, Meerman RH: Antenatal diagnosis of Potter syndrome. Obstet Gynecol 52:64S, 1978.
Miskin M: Prenatal diagnosis of renal agenesis by ultrasonography and maternal pyelography. AJR
  132:1025, 1979.
Pircon RA, Porto M, Towers CV, et al.: Ultrasound findings in pregnancies complicated by fetal triploidy.
  J Ultrasound Med 8:507, 1989.
Romero R, Cullen M, Grannum P, et al.: Antenatal diagnosis of renal anomalies with ultrasound. III.
  Bilateral renal agenesis. Am J Obstet Gynecol 151:38, 1985.
Romero R, Cullen M, Jeanty P, et al.: The diagnosis of congenital renal anomalies with ultrasound. II.
  Infantile polycystic kidney disease. Am J Obstet Gynecol 150:259, 1984.
Shih WJ, Greenbaum LD, Baro C: In utero sonogram in prune-belly syndrome. Urology 20:102, 1982.
Simpson JL, Sabbagha RE, Elias S, et al.: Failure to detect polycystic kidneys in utero by second
  trimester ultrasonography. Hum Genet 60:295, 1982.
Sirtori M, Ghidini A, Romero R, et al.: Prenatal diagnosis of sirenomelia. J Ultrasound Med 8:83,
  1989.
Sumner TE, Volberg FM, Martin JF: Real-time sonography of congenital cystic kidney disease. Urology
  20:97, 1982.

NONIMMUNE HYDROPS FETALIS

Hematologic

Comment

Anemia due to maternal acquired pure
   red cell aplasia
Anemia due to blood loss
   Fetomaternal bleeding
   Twin-to-twin transfusion
Hemolysis   Glucose-6-phosphate dehydrogenase
                                   deficiency
Hemoglobinopathy   Homozygous alpha-thalassemia

Pulmonary

Thoracic enteric duplication cyst
CCAM   Congenital cystic adenomatoid
                                  malformation

Pulmonary lymphangiectasia
Pulmonary leiomyosarcoma
Alveolar cell adenoma of the lung
Diaphragmatic hernia
Extralobar pulmonary sequestration
Enlargement of one lung
Chylothorax

Neurologic

Fetal intracranial hemorrhage
Encephalocele
Porencephaly with absent corpus
   callosum

Gastrointestinal

Neck hemangioendothelioma
Midgut volvulus
Diaphragmatic hernia
Atresia
   Esophageal with imperforate anus
   Duodenal
   Bowel
   Ileal with meconium peritonitis

Meconium peritonitis with gut
herniated into peritoneal sac
Meconium peritonitis of unknown
etiology
Duodenal diverticulum
Imperforate anus
Simulated by meconium peritonitis

Hepatic

Cirrhosis with portal hypertension
Giant cell hepatitis
Hepatic necrosis
Hemangioendothelioma of the liver

Genitourinary

Congenital nephrotic syndrome
(Finnish type)
Pelvic kidney
Hypoplastic kidney (with
microcephaly)
Urethral obstruction with renal
dysplasia
Hypoplastic uterus, imperforate
hymen, and bilateral accessory renal
arteries
Polycystic kidneys, vaginal atresia,
and hydrocolpos
Urogenital sinus, hydronephrosis, bifid
uterus, and hydrocolpos
APKD

Infectious

Coxsackievirus pancarditis
Secondary syphilis
Toxoplasmosis
Cytomegalovirus hepatitis,
myocarditis, and encephalitis
Parvovirus
Herpes simplex type I
Respiratory syncytial virus

Neoplastic

Neuroblastoma
Teratoma
Sacral

Neoplastic (Continued)

Mediastinal
Malignant
Congenital leukemia with Down
  syndrome
Hemangioendothelioma of the liver
Pulmonary leiomyosarcoma
Tuberous sclerosis

Cardiovascular

Cardiac structure
  Acute closure of foramen ovale
  A-V canal defect
    With abdominal situs inversus and
      complete heart block
    With transposition of great
      arteries
    With transposition of the great
      vessels and asplenia
    With transposition of the great
      vessels and polysplenia
    With double outlet right ventricle
      and pulmonic stenosis
    With overriding aorta,
      tracheoesophageal fistula
    With complex bradyarrhythmia,
      A-V valve insufficiency, and
      interrupted IVC
    Complete communication with
      common A-V valve
  Tetralogy of Fallot
  Absent pulmonary valve or
    pulmonary atresia
  Aortic atresia, diminutive left
    ventricle and mitral valve
  Aortic valve stenosis with mitral
    insufficiency
  Aortic arch interruption
  Tricuspid dysplasia and Ebstein's
    anomaly
  Tricuspid and pulmonary atresia
  Myocardial infarction with coronary
    artery embolus
  Intrapericardial teratoma
  Cardiac rhabdomyoma
  Myocardial tumors involving
    ventricular septum, aortic outflow,

and left atrium, not requiring
surgery
Intrauterine closure of foramen
ovale
Intrauterine closure of ductus
arteriosus
Endocardial fibroelastosis
With mitral valve insufficiency
With subaortic stenosis
VSD
ASD
With ASD and right atrial
conduction system hamartoma
With patent ductus arteriosus
With absent right hemidiaphragm
Cardiac rhythm
Atrial
Bradycardia and bradyarrhythmia
Tachycardia
Paroxysmal (PAT)
Wolff-Parkinson-White (WPW)
Flutter with block
Complete heart block
Vascular
Vena cava thrombosis
Hemangioendothelioma
Atrial calcification
Arterovenous malformation
Cerebral angioma
Metabolic
Gaucher's disease
Sialidosis
Gangliosidosis GM1
Mucopolysaccharidosis
Skeletal dysplasias
Achondroplasia
Achondrogenesis
Parenti-Fraccaro (or type I)
Langer-Saldino (or type II)
Osteogenesis imperfecta
Thanatophoric dwarfism
Short rib-polydactyly syndrome
Saldino-Noonan type
Majewski type
Asphyxiating thoracic dysplasia
Chromosomal
Triploidy

Trisomies

13
21 (Down syndrome)
E
18 (Edward's syndrome)
Translocation E
47XY + der, t(11:21) (q23:q11)mat
Abnormal chromosome 11
Mosaic 46XX/XY
Mosaic 46XY/92XXYY
45XO (Turner's syndrome)
dup(11p)

Hereditary

Pena-Shokier type I
Lethal multiple pterygium syndrome
Idiopathic
Noonan's syndrome with congenital
    heart defect

Placental

Chorioangioma

Cyr DR, Guntheroth WG, Nyberg DA, et al.: Prenatal diagnosis of an intrapericardial teratoma: A cause for nonimmune hydrops. J Ultrasound Med 7:87, 1988.

Dillard JP, Edwards DK, Leopold GR: Meconium peritonitis masquerading as fetal hydrops. J Ultrasound Med 6:49, 1987.

Etches PC, Lemons JA: Nonimmune hydrops fetalis. Report of 22 cases including their siblings. Pediatrics 64:326, 1979.

Franzek DA, Strayer SA, Hull MT, et al.: Enteric cyst as a cause of nonimmune hydrops fetalis: Fetal thoracentesis with fluid analysis. J Clin Ultrasound 17:275, 1989.

Graves GR, Baskett TF: Non-immune hydrops fetalis: Antenatal diagnosis and management. Am J Obstet Gynecol 148:563, 1984.

Holzgreve W, Curry CJR, Golbus M, et al.: Investigation of non-immune hydrops fetalis. Am J Obstet Gynecol 150:805, 1984.

McGahan JP, Schneider JM: Fetal neck hemangioendothelioma with secondary hydrops fetalis: Sonographic diagnosis. J Clin Ultrasound 14:383, 1986.

Platt LD, Collea JV, Joseph DM: Transitory fetal ascites: An ultrasound diagnosis. Am J Obstet Gynecol 132:906, 1978.

Romero R, Pilu G, Jeanty P, Ghidini A, Hobbins J: *Prenatal Diagnosis of Congenital Anomalies.* Norwalk, Conn, Appleton & Lange, 1988, pp 417-418.

Thomas CS, Leopold GR, Hilton S, et al.: Fetal hydrops associated with extralobar pulmonary sequestration. J Ultrasound Med 6:688, 1986.

Weiner C, Varner M, Pringle K, et al.: Antenatal diagnosis and palliative treatment of non-immune hydrops fetalis secondary to pulmonary extralobar sequestration. Obstet Gynecol 68:275, 1986.

Cord and Placenta

UMBILICAL CORD MASSES

	Comment
Omphalomesenteric cyst	Rare; usually in males
Allantoic cyst	Omphalocele or urachus may be associated
Hematoma	
Thrombosis of umbilical vessels	
Hemangioma of the cord	Hyperechogenic
Teratoma	
False knot	
True knot	
Transient cyst	
Vitelline duct cyst	
Mucoid degeneration of cord	Cyst-like, at cord insertion into fetus
Ectasia of umbilical vein	
Angiomyxoma	
Umbilical vein varix	

Genkins SM, Hertzberg BS, Bowie JD, et al.: Pena-Shokeir type I syndrome: In utero sonographic appearance. J Clin Ultrasound 17:56, 1989.

Ghidini A, Romero R, Eisen RN, et al.: Umbilical cord hemangioma: Prenatal identification and review of the literature. J Ultrasound Med 9:297, 1990.

Iaccarino M, Baldi F, Persico O, et al.: Ultrasonographic and pathologic study of mucoid degeneration of umbilical cord. J Clin Ultrasound 14:127, 1986.

Jauniaux E, Moscoso G, Chitty L, et al.: An angiomyxoma involving the whole length of the umbilical cord. J Ultrasound Med 9:419, 1990.

Jeanty P: Fetal and funicular vascular anomalies: Identification with prenatal US. Radiology 173:367, 1989.

Rempen A: Sonographic first-trimester diagnosis of umbilical cord cyst. J Clin Ultrasound 17:53, 1989.

Romero R, Pilu G, Jeanty P, Ghidini A, Hobbins J: *Prenatal Diagnosis of Congenital Anomalies.* Norwalk, Conn, Appleton & Lange, 1988, pp 392-395, 397, 399.

Sachs L, Fourcroy JL, Wenzel DJ, et al.: Prenatal detection of umbilical cord allantoic cyst. Radiology 145:445, 1982.

Vesce F, Guerrini P, Perri G, et al.: Ultrasonographic diagnosis of ectasia of the umbilical vein. J Clin Ultrasound 15:346, 1987.

PLACENTAL LUCENCIES

	Comment
Normal subplacental complex	
Intervillous thrombosis	
Septal cysts	
Massive subchorial thrombus	Rare; leads to abortion
Hydatidiform change	Complete mole or triploidy
Chorioangioma	
Teratoma	
Metastases	
Avillous spaces	
Maternal lakes	
Subchorial lakes	
Subchorionic fibrin deposition	
Bleeding after chorionic villous sampling	
Infarct	May not be visible at ultrasound
Mature placenta	
Hematoma	
Placenta circumvallate	Part of placenta not covered by chorion
Subchorionic thrombosis	

Almond DC, Fenton DW, Kennedy A, et al.: Ultrasonic evidence that massive subchorial thrombohematoma is an antemortem event. J Clin Ultrasound 11:49, 1983.

Cooperberg PL, Wright VJ, Carpenter CW: Ultrasonographic demonstration of a placental maternal lake. J Clin Ultrasound 7:62, 1979.

Fisher CC, Garrett W, Kossoff G: Placental aging monitored by gray scale echography. Am J Obstet Gynecol 124:483, 1976.

Hoogland HJ: *Ultrasonographic Aspects of the Placenta*. Alphen ald Rijn, The Netherlands, Stafleu, 1980.

Jauniaux E, Avni FE, Donner C, et al.: Ultrasonographic diagnosis and morphological study of placenta circumvallate. J Clin Ultrasound 17:126, 1989.

Jauniaux E, Campbell S: Fetal growth retardation with abnormal blood flows and placental sonographic lesions. J Clin Ultrasound 18:210, 1990.

Marx M, Casola G, Scheible W, et al.: The subplacental complex: Further sonographic observations. J Ultrasound Med 4:459, 1985.

Pedersen JF, Mantoni M: Prevalence and significance of subchorionic hemorrhage in threatened abortion. A sonographic study. AJR 154:535, 1990.

Pircon RA, Porto M, Towers CV, et al.: Ultrasound findings in pregnancies complicated by fetal triploidy. J Ultrasound Med 8:507, 1989.

Pozniak MA, Cullenward MJ, Zickuhr D, et al.: Venous lake bleeding: A complication of chorionic villus sampling. J Ultrasound Med 7:297, 1988.

Spirit BA, Gordon LP: Sonographic evaluation of the placenta: Importance of pathologic correlation. Radiology 176:9, 1990.

PLACENTAL MASSES

Fetal triploidy
Chorioangioma

Pircon RA, Porto M, Towers CV, et al.: Ultrasound findings in pregnancies complicated by fetal triploidy. J Ultrasound Med 8:507, 1989.
Wolfe BK, Kirk Wallace JH: Pitfall to avoid: Chorioangioma of the placenta simulating fetal tumor. J Clin Ultrasound 15:405, 1987.

ENLARGED (THICKENED) PLACENTA

Maternal diabetes
Rh disease
Infection
Triploidy
Maternal heart failure
Hydropic fetus

Crane JP, Beaver HA, Cheung SW: Antenatal ultrasound findings in fetal triploidy syndrome. J Ultrasound Med 4:519, 1985.

Fetal Size

LARGE FOR DATES

Genetic
Infant of diabetic mother

Miller JM, Kissling GE, Brown HL, et al.: In utero growth of the large-for-menstrual-age fetus. J Clin Ultrasound 17:15, 1989.

Intrauterine Membranes

	Comment
Amniotic sheets	
Chorioamnionic separation	First trimester
Amniotic band syndrome	
Harlequin ichthyosis	Thickened skin which may slough
Subchorionic hemorrhage	
Intrauterine shelves	Normal fetal anatomy excludes amniotic band syndrome

Brown DL, Felker RE, Emerson DS: Intrauterine shelves in pregnancy: Sonographic observations. AJR 153:821, 1989.

Mahoney B, Filly RA, Callen PW, et al.: The amniotic band syndrome: Antenatal sonographic diagnosis and potential pitfalls. Am J Obstet Gynecol 152:63, 1985.

Mihalko M, Lindfors KK, Grix AW, et al.: Prenatal sonographic diagnosis of harlequin ichthyosis. AJR 153:827, 1989.

Randel SB, Filly RA, Callen PW, et al.: Amniotic sheets. Radiology 166:633, 1988.

Sauerbrei EE, Pham DH: Placental abruption and subchorionic hemorrhage in the first half of pregnancy: US appearance and clinical outcome. Radiology 160:109, 1986.

PART III
PEDIATRIC

NEONATAL BRAIN

Echogenic area, region of
    germinal matrix
Echogenic areas within brain
Echogenic material within ventricle
    or cerebrospinal fluid
Cystic brain lesions
Dilated ventricles
Solid lesions
Brain calcifications

NECK

Masses

CHEST

Mediastinal masses
Extramediastinal chest pathology

STOMACH

Pyloric wall thickening

LIVER

Echogenic or hypoechoic liver
    lesions
Enlarged liver
Cysts
Bright periportal echoes (starry-sky
    liver)

GALLBLADDER

Echogenic mass
Hydrops

BILIARY TRACT

Dilatation

PANCREAS

Echogenic
Cysts

BOWEL

Wall thickening

SPLEEN

Focal echogenic abnormalities

KIDNEYS

Urinary tract dilatation, renal pelvis,
    or proximal ureter
Urinary tract dilatation, distal ureter
Multiple hypoechoic areas
Renal masses, unilateral
Renal masses, bilateral
Echogenic mass in collecting
    system
Cysts

Enlarged, unilateral
Enlarged, bilateral
Small, unilateral
Small, bilateral
Echogenic
Hyperechoic pyramids
Calcifications
Perirenal fluid

ADRENALS

Masses
Cysts

BLADDER

Wall thickening
Masses

PELVIC MASSES

Presacral
Rectovesical
Male

OVARIES AND ADNEXA

Cysts
Masses, solid or complex

TESTES, SCROTUM, AND EPIDIDYMIS

Enlarged testes
Small testes
Enlarged scrotum
Masses, extratesticular
Enlarged epididymis

Neonatal Brain

ECHOGENIC AREA, REGION OF GERMINAL MATRIX

Common

Subependymal hemorrhage
Echogenic choroid plexus

Uncommon

Normal caudothalamic groove
Periventricular leukomalacia
Nonhemorrhagic infarction
Calcification
Hamartoma

Comment

May not shadow
Especially in tuberous sclerosis

Slovis TL, Shkolnik A, Haller JO: Focal areas of increased echogenicity within the brain. J Ultrasound Med 8:31, 1989.
Siedler DE, Mahony BS, Hoddick WK, et al.: A specular reflection arising from the ventricular wall: A potential pitfall in the diagnosis of germinal matrix hemorrhage. J Ultrasound Med 4:109, 1985.

ECHOGENIC AREAS WITHIN BRAIN

Common	Comment
Normal caudothalamic groove	
Brain infarct	Especially infants on extracorporeal membranous oxygen (ECMO)
Calcification	May not shadow

Uncommon	
Tumor	
Encephalitis	
Edema from asphyxia	Especially thalamus and basal ganglia
Pseudolesion	Tangential imaging of sulcus; disappears when transducer is rotated
Hamartoma	Especially in tuberous sclerosis
AVM	
Leptomeningeal	As seen in Sturge-Weber syndrome anastomosis
Air	Air embolism

Babcock DS, Ball W: Ultrasound diagnosis and short-term prognosis of post-asphyxial encephalopathy in term infants. *Proceedings, Second Special Ross Laboratories Conference on Perinatal Intracranial Hemorrhage Syllabus*, Washington, DC, Vol. I, p 697, Dec 2-4, 1982.

Babcock DS, Han BK, Weiss RG, et al.: Brain abnormalities in infants on extracorporeal membrane oxygenation: Sonographic and CT findings. AJR 153:571, 1989.

Hertzberg BS, Pasto ME, Needleman L, et al.: Postasphyxial encephalopathy in term infants: Sonographic demonstration of increased echogenicity of the thalamus and basal ganglia. J Ultrasound Med 6:197, 1987.

Nanni GS, Kaude JV, Reeder JD: Ischemic brain infarct in a neonate: Ultrasound diagnosis and follow-up. J Clin Ultrasound 12:229, 1984.

Reeder JD, Sanders RC: Ventriculitis in the neonate: Recognition by sonography. AJNR 4:37, 1983.

Siedler DE, Mahony BS, Hoddick WK, et al.: A specular reflection arising from the ventricular wall: A potential pitfall in the diagnosis of germinal matrix hemorrhage. J Ultrasound Med 4:109, 1985.

Slovis TL, Shkolnik A, Haller JO: Focal areas of increased echogenicity within the brain. J Ultrasound Med 8:31, 1989.

Widder DJ, Davis KR, Taveras JM: Assessment of ventricular shunt patency by sonography: A new noninvasive test. AJR 147:353, 1986.

ECHOGENIC MATERIAL WITHIN VENTRICLE OR CEREBROSPINAL FLUID

Common

Intraventricular hemorrhage

Uncommon

Meningitis
Ventriculitis
Air

Comment

In air embolization or in shunt failure

Vachon L, Mikity V: Computed tomography and ultrasound in purulent ventriculitis. J Ultrasound Med 6:269, 1987.
Widder DJ, Davis KR, Taveras JM: Assessment of ventricular shunt patency by sonography: A new noninvasive test. AJR 147:353, 1986.

CYSTIC BRAIN LESIONS

Common

Porencephalic cysts

Uncommon

Schizencephaly
Dandy-Walker cysts
Arachnoid cysts
Ventricular cysts
Arteriovenous malformations
Vein of Galen aneurysms
Alobar holoprosencephaly
Agenesis of corpus callosum with
    midline cyst

McGahan JP, Ellis W, Lindfors KK, et al.: Congenital cerebrospinal fluid-containing intracranial abnormalities: A sonographic classification. J Clin Ultrasound 16:531, 1988.

DILATED VENTRICLES

Common

Hydrocephalus
  Obstructing mass
  Aqueductal stenosis
  Obstruction over convexities
  Obstruction at level of superior
    sagittal sinus

Uncommon

Semilobar holoprosencephaly
After hemorrhage
Associated with meningomyelocele
Dandy-Walker cyst
Ventriculitis
Simulated by hydranencephaly

Britton CA: Semilobar holoprosencephaly with associated Arnold-Chiari variant. J Clin Ultrasound 17:374, 1989.

Sims ME, Halterman G, Jasani N, et al.: Indications for routine cranial ultrasound scanning in the nursery. J Clin Ultrasound 14:443, 1986.

Vachon L, Mikity V: Computed tomography and ultrasound in purulent ventriculitis. J Ultrasound Med 6:269, 1987.

SOLID LESIONS

	Comment
Lipoma of corpus callosum	Solid; echogenic; midline
Hamartoma	
Glioma	
Ependymoma	Brainstem mass
Astrocytoma	

Boechat MI, Kangarloo H, Diament MJ, et al.: Lipoma of the corpus callosum: Sonographic appearance. J Clin Ultrasound 11:447, 1983.

BRAIN CALCIFICATIONS

Common	Comment
TORCH	Toxoplasmosis, other (viruses), rubella, CMV, herpes

Uncommon

AIDS
Down syndrome
Familial encephalopathies
Radiation
Carbon monoxide poisoning
Lead poisoning
Vitamin D intoxication
Hyperparathyroidism

Belman AL, Lantos G, Horoupian D, et al.: AIDS: Calcification of the basal ganglia in infants and children. Neurology 36:1192, 1986.

Neck

MASSES

Common	Comment
Lymphadenopathy	Solid and/or heterogeneous

Uncommon

Thyroglossal duct cyst
Thyroid lesion
  Adenoma
  Carcinoma
  Ectopic thyroid tissue
  Follicular cysts
Metastases
Lymphoma
Neurofibroma
Hemangioma   Cystic: complex or solid

Sherman NH, Rosenberg HK, Heyman S, et al.: Ultrasound evaluation of neck masses in children. J Ultrasound Med 4:127, 1985.

Chest

MEDIASTINAL MASSES

Common	Comment
Neuroblastoma	Ganglioneuroma
Normal thymus	Can be homogeneously echogenic or anechoic

Uncommon	
Neurofibroma	
Bronchogenic cysts	
Neurenteric cysts	
Duplication cysts	
Teratomas/dermoids	Can be solid or cystic or hypoechoic
Cystic hygroma	
Lipoma	
Thymoma	
Hemangioma	
Sarcoma of thymus	
Lymphoma/leukemia	Variable; mainly solid, homogeneous masses
Thymic cysts	

Miller JH, Reid BS, Kemberling CR: Water-path ultrasound of chest disease in children. Radiol 152:401, 1984.

Ries T, Currarino G, Nikaidoh H, et al.: Real-time ultrasonography of subcarinal bronchogenic cysts in two children. Radiology 145:121, 1982.

Rudick MG, Wood BP: The use of ultrasound in the diagnosis of a large thymic cyst. Pediatr Radiol 10:113, 1980.

Shkolnik A, Williams J: The chest, in Haller JO, Shkolnik A (eds): *Ultrasound in Pediatrics.* New York, Churchill Livingstone, 1981, pp 28-55.

Sumner TE, Volberg FM, Kiser PE, et al.: Mediastinal cystic hygroma in children. Pediatr Radiol 11:160, 1981.

EXTRAMEDIASTINAL CHEST PATHOLOGY

Common	Comment
Pleural effusion	
Pulmonary consolidations/atelectasis	Homogeneous and more echogenic than liver
Pulmonary fibrosis	

Uncommon

Congenital cysts
  Congenital lung cyst
  Peripheral bronchogenic cyst
Cystic adenomatoid malformation
False aneurysm
Teratoma
Lymphoma
Diaphragmatic hernia
Pulmonary sequestration
Granulomas
Pseudotumors
Bronchial adenomas
Pulmonary blastomas
Bronchogenic carcinoma

Hartenberg MA, Brewer WH: Cystic adenomatoid malformation of the lung: Identification by sonography. AJR 140:694, 1983.

Jaffe MH, Bank ER, Silver TM, et al.: Pulmonary sequestration: Ultrasonic appearance. J Clin Ultrasound 10:294, 1982.

O'Laughlin MP, Huhta JC, Murphy DJ: Ultrasound examination of extracardiac chest masses in children: Doppler diagnosis of a vascular etiology. J Ultrasound Med 6:151, 1987.

West MS, Donaldson JS, Shkolnik A: Pulmonary sequestration: Diagnosis by ultrasound. J Ultrasound Med 8:125, 1989.

Stomach

PYLORIC WALL THICKENING

Common

Hypertrophic pyloric stenosis

Comment

Uncommon

Chronic granulomatous disease of
  childhood
Ectopic pancreas
Hematoma
Peptic ulcer disease
Gastritis
Duplication cyst
Ménétrier's disease
Caustic agent ingestion
Crohn's disease

Bisset RAL, Gupta SC: Hypertrophic pyloric stenosis: Ultrasonic appearances in a small baby. Pediatr Radiol 18:405, 1988.

Blumhagen JD, Maclin L, Krauter D, et al.: Sonographic diagnosis of hypertrophic pyloric stenosis. AJR 150:1367, 1988.

Kofoed P-EL, Høst A, Elle B, et al.: Hypertrophic pyloric stenosis: Determination of muscle dimensions by ultrasound. Br J Radiol 61:19, 1988.

Weiskittel DA, Leary DL, Blane CE: Ultrasound diagnosis of evolving pyloric stenosis. Gastrointest Radiol 14:22, 1989.

Westra SJ, de Groot CJ, Smits NJ, et al.: Hypertrophic pyloric stenosis: Use of the pyloric volume measurement in early US diagnosis. Radiology 172:615, 1989.

Liver

ECHOGENIC OR HYPOECHOIC LIVER LESIONS

Common	Comment
Metastases	
Neuroblastoma	Usually echogenic
Hodgkin's disease	
Lymphoma	More often gives focal masses in pediatrics
Cysts	
Focal nodular hyperplasia	
Adenoma	
Regenerating nodules	
Sarcoma, undifferentiated	
Rhabdomyosarcoma	
Angiosarcoma	
Fibrosarcoma	
Leiomyosarcoma	
Teratocarcinoma	
Hemangioma	Most common benign tumor
Capillary	
Cavernous	
Infection	
Abscess	

Uncommon

Hepatoblastoma	First 3 years of life
Hepatoma	Usually after 5 to 6 years of age
Biliary rhabdomyosarcoma	Before age 5
Mesenchymal hamartoma	
Teratoma	
Hamartoma	
Cavernous transformation portal vein	
Calcified ductus venosus	In neonates, curvilinear density
Fatty infiltration	Malnutrition, hyperalimentation, and steroids

Frider B, Marín AM, Goldberg A: Ultrasonographic diagnosis of portal vein cavernous transformation in children. J Ultrasound Med 8:445, 1989.

Jackson FI, Lalani Z: Ultrasound in the diagnosis of lymphoma: A review. J Clin Ultrasound 17:145, 1989.

Kenney IJ, Hendry GMA, Mackinlay GA: Spontaneous regression of mesenchymal hamartoma: Observations using ultrasound. J Clin Ultrasound 14:72, 1986.

Klein MA, Slovis TL, Chang CH, et al.: Sonographic and Doppler features of infantile hepatic hemangiomas with pathologic correlation. J Ultrasound Med 9:619, 1990.

Kraudel K, Williams CH: Ultrasound case report of hepatic teratoma in newborn. J Clin Ultrasound 12:98, 1984.

Marks F, Thomas P, Lustig I, et al.: In utero sonographic description of a fetal liver adenoma. J Ultrasound Med 9:119, 1990.

Rizzo AJ, Haller JO, Mulvihill DM, et al.: Calcification of the ductus venosus: A cause of right upper quadrant calcification in the newborn. Radiology 173:89, 1989.

Williams AG, Sheward SE: Ultrasound appearance of biliary rhabdomyosarcoma. J Clin Ultrasound 14:63, 1986.

ENLARGED LIVER

Common	*Comment*
Hepatitis	
Metastases	
Heart failure	

Uncommon	
Lymphoma	
Mesenchymal hamartoma	Usually cystic
Hemangioendothelioma	Most before 6 months; have heart failure
Cavernous hemangioma	Rare in infants
Teratoma	
Neonatal hepatitis	Usually normal-sized liver
Wolman's disease	Hereditary
Heart failure	
Extramedullary hematopoiesis	
Rhabdomyosarcoma	

Jackson FI, Lalani Z: Ultrasound in the diagnosis of lymphoma: A review. J Clin Ultrasound 17:145, 1989.

Kenney IJ, Hendry GMA, Mackinlay GA: Spontaneous regression of mesenchymal hamartoma: Observations using ultrasound. J Clin Ultrasound 14:72, 1986.

Kraudel K, Williams CH: Ultrasound case report of hepatic teratoma in newborn. J Clin Ultrasound 12:98, 1984.

CYSTS

Congenital
With APKD
Echinococcus
Amebic
Abscess
Choledochal cyst
Biloma
Ectopic gallbladder

Athey PA, Lauderman JA, King DE: Massive congenital solitary nonparasitic cyst of the liver in infancy. J Ultrasound Med 5:585, 1986.

Austin RM, Sussman S, McArdle CR, et al.: Case report. Computed tomographic and ultrasound appearances of a solitary intrahepatic choledochal cyst. Clin Radiol 37:149, 1986.

Bezzi M, Teggi A, De Rosa F, et al.: Abdominal hydatid disease: US findings during medical treatment. Radiology 162:91, 1987.

Didier D, Weiler S, Rohmer P, et al.: Hepatic alveolar echinococcosis: Correlative US and CT study. Radiology 154:179, 1985.

Levine E, Cook LT, Grantham JJ: Liver cysts in autosomal-dominant polycystic kidney disease: Clinical and computed tomographic study. AJR 145:229, 1985.

BRIGHT PERIPORTAL ECHOES (STARRY-SKY LIVER)

Hepatitis
Kaposi's sarcoma
Leukemia
CMV infection
Biliary atresia
Cholangitis
Cystic fibrosis
Mononucleosis
Right heart failure

Giorgio A, Amoroso P, Fico P, et al.: Ultrasound evaluation of uncomplicated and complicated acute viral hepatitis. J Clin Ultrasound 14:675, 1986.

Lee S: Hepatic oil embolism following lymphangiography. J Ultrasound Med 4:357, 1985.

Luburich P, Bru C, Ayuso MC, et al.: Hepatic Kaposi sarcoma in AIDS: US and CT findings. Radiology 175:172, 1990.

Needleman L, Kurtz A, Rifkin M, et al.: Sonography of diffuse benign liver disease: Accuracy of pattern recognition and grading. AJR 146:1011, 1986.

Rak K, Hopper KD, Parker SH: The "starry sky" liver with Burkitt's lymphoma. J Ultrasound Med 7:279, 1988.

Gallbladder

ECHOGENIC MASS

Common

Stones

Comment

Associated with hemolytic states, cystic fibrosis, biliary tract malformations, obesity, Wilson's disease, total parenteral nutrition (TPN), furosemide in infants, malabsorption, hepatitis, and prolonged fast

Uncommon

Pus
Blood
Worms
Ectopic pancreas
Ectopic gastric tissue

Benjamin D: Cholelithiasis in infants: The role of total parenteral nutrition and gastrointestinal dysfunction. J Pediatr Surg 17:386, 1982.

Ramey SL, Williams JL: Nephrolithiasis and cholelithiasis in a premature infant. J Clin Ultrasound 14:203, 1986.

HYDROPS

Comment

Biliary obstruction
Acute or chronic cholecystitis
Mucocutaneous lymph node syndrome   Also known as Kawasaki disease
Acalculous cholecystitis
Typhoid fever

Bradford BF, Reid B, Weinstein BJ, et al.: Ultrasonographic evaluation of the gallbladder in mucocutaneous lymph node syndrome. Radiology 142:381, 1982.

Chamberlain JW, Hight DW: Acute hydrops of the gallbladder in childhood. Surgery 68:899, 1970.

Chandnani PC, Chabria PB, Perrell CV, et al.: Ultrasound as an aid in the diagnosis of hydrops of the gallbladder. JAMA 237:996, 1977.

Cohen EK, Stringer DA, Smith CR, et al.: Hydrops of the gallbladder in typhoid fever as demonstrated by sonography. J Clin Ultrasound 14:633, 1986.

Kumari S, Lee WJ, Baron MG: Hydrops of the gallbladder in a child: Diagnosis by ultrasonography. Pediatrics 63:295, 1979.

Magilavy DB, Speert P, Silver TM, et al.: Mucocutaneous lymph node syndrome: Report of two cases complicated by gallbladder hydrops and diagnosed by ultrasound. Pediatrics 61:699, 1978.

Slovis TL, Hight DW, Philippart AI, et al.: Sonography in the diagnosis and management of hydrops of the gallbladder in children with mucocutaneous lymph node syndrome. Pediatrics 65:789, 1980.

Sty JR, Starshak RJ, Gorenstein L: Gallbladder perforation in a case of Kawasaki disease: Image correlation. J Clin Ultrasound 11:381, 1983.

Wicks JD, Silver TM, Bree RL: Giant cystic abdominal masses in children and adolescents: Ultrasonic differential diagnosis. Am J Roentgenol 130:853, 1978.

Biliary Tract

DILATATION

	Comment
Ductal ectasia	Poor prognosis
Congenital hepatic fibrosis with biliary ectasia	
Caroli's disease	Segmental dilatation; no fibrosis
Choledochal cyst	Extrahepatic ducts cystically dilated
Biliary atresia	
Obstruction of common bile duct	
Common duct stone	
Lymphadenopathy	
Biliary rhabdomyosarcoma	Usually before age 5
Pancreatitis	
Choledochal cysts	

Williams AG, Sheward SE: Ultrasound appearance of biliary rhabdomyosarcoma. J Clin Ultrasound 14:63, 1986.

Pancreas

ECHOGENIC

	Comment
Cystic fibrosis	Fatty infiltration
Obesity	Fatty infiltration
Chronic pancreatitis	
Steroids	
Hereditary pancreatitis	

Gupta AK, Arenson A-M, McKee JD, et al.: Effect of steroid ingestion on pancreatic echogenicity. J Clin Ultrasound 15:171, 1987.

So CB, Cooperberg PL, Gibney RG, et al.: Sonographic findings in pancreatic lipomatosis. AJR 149:67, 1987.

CYSTS

	Comment
Pseudocyst	Usually posttraumatic in children
APKD	
Abscess	
Hematoma	

Bloom RA, Abu-Dalu K, Pollak D: Spontaneous resolution of a large pancreatic pseudocyst in a child. J Clin Ultrasound 11:37, 1983.

Bowel

WALL THICKENING

Crohn's disease
Typhlitis
Necrotizing enterocolitis
Amebic colitis
Intussusception
Ménétrier's disease

Hematoma in wall

Comment

Seen in leukemia
Seen in neonates

Protein losing enteropathy plus
  hypertrophic gastropathy
Child abuse should be considered in
  younger age groups

Burke LF, Clarke E: Ileocolic intussusception: A case report. J Clin Ultrasound 5:346, 1977.
Gassner I, Strasser K, Bart G, et al.: Sonographic appearance of Ménétrier's disease in a child. J Ultrasound Med 9:537, 1990.
Hernanz-Schulman M, Genieser NB, Ambrosino M: Sonographic diagnosis of intramural duodenal hematoma. J Ultrasound Med 8:273, 1989.
Hussain S, Dinshaw H: Ultrasonography in amebic colitis. J Ultrasound Med 9:385, 1990.
Montali G, Groce F, De Pra L, et al.: Intussusception of the bowel: A sonographic pattern. Br J Radiol 56:621, 1983.
Patel U, Leonidas JC, Furie D: Sonographic detection of necrotizing enterocolitis in infancy. J Ultrasound Med 9:673, 1990.
Rodgers B, Seibert JJ: Unusual combination of an appendicolith in a leukemic patient with typhlitis — Ultrasound diagnosis. J Clin Ultrasound 18:191, 1990.
Verbank JJ, Rutgeerts LJ, Donterlunge PH, et al.: Sonographic and pathologic correlations in intussusception of the bowel. J Clin Ultrasound 14:393, 1986.

Spleen

FOCAL ECHOGENIC ABNORMALITIES

	Comment
Cysts	May be congenital or acquired
Abscesses	May be seen with endocarditis
Hematomas	
Infarction	
Lymphoma	
Metastases	
Cat-scratch fever	

Cox F, Perlman S, Sathyanarayana: Splenic abscesses in cat scratch disease: Sonographic diagnosis and follow-up. J Clin Ultrasound 17:511, 1989.

KIDNEYS

URINARY TRACT DILATATION, RENAL PELVIS, OR PROXIMAL URETER

Common

UPJ obstruction

Reflux
Dilated nonobstructed system
Distended bladder
Extrarenal pelvis

Uncommon

Overhydration
Obstruction distally
After diuretics or contrast
Flaccid system due to infection
After relief of obstruction
Megacalyces
Papillary necrosis
Solitary kidney
Retrocaval ureter
Prune-belly syndrome

Comment

Most common congenital obstruction;
often bilateral

URINARY TRACT DILATATION, DISTAL URETER

Common

Reflux
Dilated nonobstructed system
Overdistended bladder

Uncommon

UVJ obstruction
Primary mega-ureter

Overhydration
Prune-belly syndrome
Bladder outlet obstruction

Comment

Usually males; left sided; 20%
bilateral

MULTIPLE HYPOECHOIC AREAS

Common	*Comment*
Simple cysts	Especially in IPKD
Obstructed kidney	

Uncommon

Lymphoma of kidneys	
Congenital AVMs	
Multilocular cystic nephromas	
Metastases	
Multiple infarcts	
Multicystic dysplastic kidney	
Lymphangioma of kidneys	May have multiple, tiny cysts
Abscesses	

Blumhagen JD, Wood BJ, Rosenbaum DM: Sonographic evaluation of abdominal lymphangiomas in children. J Ultrasound Med 6:487, 1987.

RENAL MASSES, UNILATERAL

Common	Comment
Focal bacterial nephritis (lobar nephronia)	
Wilms' tumor	
Simple cyst	Unifocal, cystic characteristics
Obstructed duplicated system	

Uncommon	
Hamartoma	
Xanthogranulomatous pyelonephritis (tumefactive)	Associated with stones
Nephroblastomatosis	Precursor to Wilms' tumor
Metastases	
Abscess	
Multilocular cystic nephroma	Unifocal mass; echogenic and isoechoic components are present
Hemangioma	
Lymphangioma	
Compound renal pyramid	Causes hypoechoic area
Crossed fused ectopia	Look in other renal fossa
Fused supernumerary kidney	
Hematoma	
Leukemic infiltrate	
Neurofibroma	
Mesoblastic nephroma	
Rhabdomyosarcoma	
Leiomyosarcoma	
Angiomyolipoma	Should have fat in lesion
Pseudotumors	
Clear-cell sarcoma of kidney	

Ambrosino MM, Hernanz-Schulman M, Horii SC, et al.: Prenatal diagnosis of nephroblastomatosis in two siblings. J Ultrasound Med 9:49, 1990.

Blumhagen JD, Wood BJ, Rosenbaum DM: Sonographic evaluation of abdominal lymphangiomas in children. J Ultrasound Med 6:487, 1987.

Jones BE, Hoffer FA, Teele RL, et al.: The compound renal pyramid: A normal hypoechoic region on the pediatric sonogram. J Ultrasound Med 6:515, 1987.

Lubat E, Hernanz-Schulman M, Genieser NB, et al.: Sonography of the simple and complicated ipsilateral fused kidney. J Ultrasound Med 8:109, 1989.

RENAL MASSES, BILATERAL

	Comment
Mesoblastic nephroma (fetal renal hamartoma)	Indistinguishable from Wilms' tumor
Wilms' tumor	
APKD	
Metastases	
Hamartomas	Especially in tuberous sclerosis

ECHOGENIC MASS IN COLLECTING SYSTEM

	Comment
Stone	
Teflon from Sting procedure	Teflon injected to treat reflux
Fungus balls	
Clot	
Pyonephrosis	
Neurofibroma	
Lymphoma	
Hematoma	
Normal pyramid in hydronephrotic calyx	
Sloughed pyramid	In papillary necrosis

Giuliano CT, Cohen HL, Haller JO, et al.: The Sting procedure and its complications: Sonographic evaluation. J Clin Ultrasound 18:415, 1990.

Schmitt GH, Hsu AS: Renal fungus balls: Diagnosis by ultrasound and percutaneous antegrade pyelography and brush biopsy in a premature infant. J Ultrasound Med 4:155, 1985.

CYSTS

Common	Comment
Multicystic dysplastic kidney	Most common abdominal mass in neonate; one third with obstruction of other kidney
Simple cysts	Cortical location
Obstructed upper pole of duplicated system	

Uncommon

Posterior urethral values	Cause hydronephrosis
IPKD	Small cysts; big kidneys
APKD	Increased neurofibromatosis; carcinoma of kidney; berry aneurysms
Associated with trisomy syndromes	Small cysts; trisomy 13 and 18 and triploidy
Cortical cysts with tuberous sclerosis	Also have angiomyolipomas
Multilocular cysts	May be hamartomas
Cystic Wilms' tumor	
Medullary sponge kidney	Medullary cysts measuring 1 to 3 mm
Calyceal diverticulum	
Zellweger syndrome	
Lawrence-Moon-Bardet-Biedl syndrome	
Jeune's syndrome	
Lymphangioma of kidney	
Acquired cysts of dialysis	

Blumhagen JD, Wood BJ, Rosenbaum DM: Sonographic evaluation of abdominal lymphangiomas in children. J Ultrasound Med 6:487, 1987.

Luisiri A, Sotelo-Avila C, Silberstein MJ, et al.: Sonography of the Zellweger syndrome. J Ultrasound Med 7:169, 1988.

Pretorius DH, Lee ME, Manco-Johnson ML, et al.: Diagnosis of autosomal dominant polycystic kidney disease in utero and in the young infant. J Ultrasound Med 6:249, 1987.

ENLARGED, UNILATERAL

Common

	Comment
Pyelonephritis, acute	May be hypoechoic
Multicystic dysplastic kidney complex	Cluster-of-grapes appearance; no sinus; common in infants
Obstruction	Congenital UPJ obstruction most common cause of obstruction
Compensatory hypertrophy	

Uncommon

Renal vein thrombosis	Kidney may be hypoechoic early and echogenic late; indistinct cortical medullary junction
Hamartoma	Common in tuberous sclerosis; fat in lesion is echogenic
Mass obstructing inferior vena cava or renal vein	
Arterial infarction	May be hypoechoic or echogenic
Duplicated collecting system	
Xanthogranulomatous pyelonephritis	Usually has calculus and obstructed kidney; may appear as multiple masses
Wilms' tumor	
Metastases	Melanoma; leukemia
Abscess	Unifocal mass
Simple cyst	Unifocal mass with cystic characteristics
Multilocular cystic nephroma	Unifocal mass with echogenic and isoechoic components
Congenital AVMs	Cluster of anechoic structures
Congenital hemihypertrophy	

Davidson AJ: *Radiology of the Kidney.* Philadelphia, WB Saunders, 1985.

ENLARGED, BILATERAL

Common	Comment
Multicystic dysplastic kidney with UPJ obstruction on other side	
Glomerulonephritis, acute	
Bilateral obstruction	
Bilateral duplication	
Acute tubular necrosis	May be hypoechoic or hyperechoic

Uncommon	
Bilateral pyelonephritis	Sometimes hypoechoic
Renal vein thrombosis, bilateral	Usually unilateral
Inferior vena caval thrombosis	
Posterior urethral valves with hydronephrosis	
Wilms' tumor	
Fabry's disease	Large prior to renal failure
Early in diabetes mellitus	
Hyperalimentation	
Associated with cirrhosis	
Response to contrast material	
Response to diuretics	
Leukemia	Smooth enlargement
Hodgkin's disease and lymphoma	Usually with multiple masses
Acute cortical necrosis	Usually in dehydrated patients
Acquired cystic disease of dialysis	
APKD	Cysts may not be seen early in course
IPKD	May not resolve cysts
Congenital nephrotic syndrome, Finnish type	Kidneys are echogenic
Membranous glomerulonephritis	
Lupus erythematosus	
Allergic angitis	
Goodpasture's syndrome	
Henoch-Schönlein purpura	
Thrombotic thrombocytopenic purpura	
Glomerulonephritis of SBE	
Acute interstitial nephritis	
Homozygous-S disease	
Hemophilia	
Beckwith-Wiedemann syndrome	
Gigantism	

Alkrinawi S, Gradus DBE, Goldstein J, et al.: Ultrasonographic pattern of congenital nephrotic syndrome of Finnish type. J Clin Ultrasound 17:443, 1989.

Davidson AJ: *Radiology of the Kidney*. Philadelphia, WB Saunders, 1985.

Pretorius DH, Lee E, Manco-Johnson ML, et al.: Diagnosis of autosomal dominant polycystic kidney disease in utero and in the young infant. J Ultrasound Med 6:249, 1987.

SMALL, UNILATERAL

Common	*Comment*
Reflux nephropathy	Usually associated scars
Congenital hypoplasia	
Postobstructive atrophy	

Uncommon

Infarction	Scar may be hyperechoic
Ischemia	
After radiation therapy	
Postinfectious atrophy	
Postrenal vein thrombosis	

Davidson AJ: *Radiology of the Kidney*. Philadelphia, WB Saunders, 1985.

SMALL, BILATERAL

Common	*Comment*
Chronic glomerulonephritis	
Postobstructive atrophy	
Reflux atrophy	

Uncommon

Emboli	
Hypotension	
Papillary necrosis	
Hereditary chronic nephritis (Alport's syndrome)	
Medullary cystic disease	Usually can see the cysts
Bartter's syndrome	Decreased potassium; growth failure
Amyloidosis	
Radiation nephritis	
Postinflammatory atrophy	
Postrenal vein thrombosis	Usually unilateral
Arteriosclerosis	
Hypertensive nephrosclerosis	

Davidson AJ: *Radiology of the Kidney*. Philadelphia, WB Saunders, 1985.
Strauss S, Robinson G, Lotan D, et al.: Renal sonography in Bartter syndrome. J Ultrasound Med 6:265, 1987.

ECHOGENIC

Common

	Comment
Normal in neonates and young infants	
Acute and chronic glomerulonephritis	
Acute tubular necrosis	Usually not echogenic

Uncommon

Pyelonephritis	Acute or chronic
Multicystic dysplastic kidney	
Hypertensive nephropathy	
Diabetic nephrosclerosis	
Leukemia	Usually not echogenic
Renal artery stenosis	
Nephrotic syndrome	
Renal dysplasia	
Nephrocalcinosis	
Wilms' tumor	
Angiomyolipoma	
IPKD	
Renal vein thrombosis	Only in some stages; may show punctate increase in echoes
Burkitt's lymphoma	May be secondary to uric acid nephropathy in this disease
Wegener's syndrome	
Chronic renal failure	
Renal dysplasia	
Long-term furosemide (Lasix) in premature infants	Gives nephrocalcinosis
Bartter's syndrome	Decreased potassium; growth failure
Lymphangioma	
Acute cortical necrosis	Calcified, echogenic cortex
Congenital nephrotic syndrome, Finnish type	Kidneys are enlarged
Henoch-Schönlein disease	
Sickle cell glomerulonephropathy	
Hemolytic uremic syndrome	
Glomerulonephritis	Reported in acute mesangial proliferative type
Transient nephromegaly of newborn	
Radiocontrast nephropathy	
Story's disease	
Lymphoma of kidneys	
Primary hyperoxaluria	
Glycogen storage disease	
Lowe's syndrome	

Alkrinawi S, Gradus DBE, Goldstein J, et al.: Ultrasonographic pattern of congenital nephrotic syndrome of Finnish type. J Clin Ultrasound 17:443, 1989.

Avner E, Ellis D, Jaffe R, et al.: Neonatal radiocontrast nephropathy simulating infantile polycystic kidney disease. Pediatrics 100:85, 1982.

Blumhagen JD, Wood BJ, Rosenbaum DM: Sonographic evaluation of abdominal lymphangiomas in children. J Ultrasound Med 6:487, 1987.

Brenbridge AN, Chevalier RL, Kaiser DL: Increased renal cortical echogenicity in pediatric renal disease: Histopathologic correlations. J Clin Ultrasound 14:595, 1986.

Choyke PL, Grant EG, Hoffer FA, et al.: Cortical echogenicity in the hemolytic uremic syndrome: Clinical correlation. J Ultrasound Med 7:439, 1988.

Evans JB, Shapeero LG, Roscelli JD: Infantile glomerulonephritis mimicking polycystic kidney disease. J Ultrasound Med 7:29, 1988.

Rodis JF, Vintzileos AM, Campbell WA, et al.: Intrauterine fetal growth in discordant twin gestations. J Ultrasound Med 9:443, 1990.

Stapleton FB, Hilton S, Wilcox J, et al.: Transient nephromegaly simulating infantile polycystic disease of the kidneys. Pediatrics 67:554, 1981.

Strauss S, Robinson G, Lotan D, et al.: Renal sonography in Bartter syndrome. J Ultrasound Med 6:265, 1987.

Sty JR, Starshak RJ, Hubbard AM: Acute renal cortical necrosis in hemolytic uremic syndrome. J Clin Ultrasound 11:175, 1983.

HYPERECHOIC PYRAMIDS

Common

Furosemide
Long-term steroids
Excess vitamin D
Bartter's syndrome
Transient renal insufficiency of infancy
Sickle hemoglobinopathies
Hyperparathyroidism

Uncommon

Renal tubular acidosis
Williams syndrome
Medullary sponge kidney
Achondroplasia
Hurler's disease
Dysgerminoma
Papillary necrosis
Neutrophil adherence glycoprotein
    deficiency
Prolonged immobilization
Idiopathic hypercalciuria

Schultz PK, Strife JL, Strife CF, McDaniel JD: Hyperechoic renal medullary pyramids in infants and children. Radiology 181:163-167, 1991.

CALCIFICATIONS

Common	Comment
Furosemide (Lasix) in infants	May be within collecting system and within pyramids
Stones	

Uncommon

Williams syndrome	Frequent cardiac abnormalities
Infants on TPN	Causes hypercalciuria; has led to stones in collecting system
Acute cortical necrosis	Echogenic calcified cortex
Nephroblastomatosis	Reported prenatally
Tuberculosis	
Renal tubular acidosis	
Hyperparathyroidism	
Papillary necrosis	
Hypervitaminosis D	
Wilms' tumor	10% calcify
Renal cortical necrosis	
End-stage multicystic dysplasia	
Xanthogranulomatous pyelonephritis	

Adelman RD, Abern SB, Merten D, et al.: Hypercalciuria with nephrolithiasis: A complication of total parenteral nutrition. Pediatrics 59:473, 1977.

Ambrosino MM, Hernanz-Schulman M, Horii SC, et al.: Prenatal diagnosis of nephroblastomatosis in two siblings. J Ultrasound Med 9:49, 1990.

Behan M, Martin EC, Muecke EC, et al.: Myelolipoma of the adrenal: Two cases with ultrasound and CT findings. Am J Roentgenol 129:993, 1977.

Hartmann DS, Goldman SM, Friedman AC, et al.: Angiomyolipoma: Ultrasonic-pathologic correlation. Radiology 139:451, 1981.

Jantarasami T, Larew M, Kao SCS, et al.: Ultrasound demonstration of nephrocalcinosis in William's syndrome. J Clin Ultrasound 17:533, 1989.

Lee TG, Henderson SC, Freeny PC, et al.: Ultrasound findings of renal angiomyolipoma. J Clin Ultrasound 6:150, 1978.

Ramey SL, Williams JL: Nephrolithiasis and cholelithiasis in a premature infant. J Clin Ultrasound 14:203, 1986.

Sty JR, Starshak RJ, Hubbard AM: Acute renal cortical necrosis in hemolytic uremic syndrome. J Clin Ultrasound 11:175, 1983.

PERIRENAL FLUID

Common

After trauma
Spontaneous decompression of
  obstructed system

Uncommon

After percutaneous stone removal
Infected kidney
Sonolucent rim in IPKD
Urinoma
Lymphocele
Perinephric abscess
Herniated bowel
Pancreatic pseudocysts
After percutaneous nephrostomy

Currarino G, Stannard MW, Rutledge JC: The sonolucent cortical rim in infantile polycystic kidneys: Histologic correlation. J Ultrasound Med 8:571, 1989.
Ivory CM, Dubbins PA, Wells IP, et al.: Ultrasound assessment of local complications of percutaneous renal stone removal. J Clin Ultrasound 17:345, 1989.

Adrenals

MASSES

Common	Comment
Hemorrhage	15% bilateral; hypoechoic to echogenic
Neuroblastoma	Most common tumor of infancy and childhood
Normal before 1 year	Adrenals are large in neonates; especially prominent with renal genesis

Uncommon

Hyperplasia	Usually bilateral
Adenoma	
Pheochromocytoma	
Abscess	
Urinoma	
Renal agenesis	
Adrenocortical carcinoma	
Wolman's disease	Large calcified glands
21-Hydroxylase deficiency	Bilateral enlargement in some
Adrenal cyst	
Tuberculosis	
Carcinoma	

Artigas JLR, Niclewiez ED, Silva A, et al.: Congenital adrenal cortical carcinomas. J Pediatr Surg 11:247, 1976.

Atkinson GO Jr, Kodroff MB, Gay BB Jr, et al.: Adrenal abscess in the neonate. Radiology 155:101, 1985.

Daneman A, Chan HSL, Martin DJ: Adrenal carcinoma and adenoma in children: A review of 17 cases. Pediatr Radiol 13:11, 1983.

Davies RP, Lam AH: Adrenocortical neoplasm in children. J Ultrasound Med 6:325, 1987.

Dutton RV: Wolman's disease. Ultrasound and CT diagnosis. Pediatr Radiol 15:144, 1985.

Kangarloo H, Diament MJ, Gold RH, et al.: Sonography of adrenal glands in neonates and children: Changes in appearance with age. J Clin Ultrasound 14:43, 1986.

Menzel D, Hauffa BP: Changes in size and sonographic characteristics of the adrenal glands during the first year of life and the sonographic diagnosis of adrenal hyperplasia in infants with 21-hydroxylase deficiency. J Clin Ultrasound 18:619, 1990.

Visconti EB, Peters RW, Cangir A, et al.: Unusual case of adrenal cortical carcinoma in a female infant. Arch Dis Child 53:324, 1978.

Wu, CC: Sonographic spectrum of neonatal adrenal hemorrhage: Report of a case simulating solid tumor. J Clin Ultrasound 17:45, 1989.

CYSTS

Resolving adrenal hemorrhage
Adrenal abscess
Congenital adrenal cyst

Atkinson GO Jr, Kodroff MB, Gay BB Jr, et al.: Adrenal abscess in the neonate. Radiology 155:101, 1985.
Wu CC: Sonographic spectrum of neonatal adrenal hemorrhage: Report of a case simulating solid tumor. J Clin Ultrasound 17:45, 1989.

Bladder

WALL THICKENING

Common	Comment
Cystitis	
Neurogenic bladder	
Normal in partially empty bladder	

Uncommon

Cyclophosphamide-induced hemorrhagic cystitis	
Outlet obstruction	
Neurofibromatosis	
Crohn's disease involvement of bladder	Look for adherent bowel
Rhabdomyosarcoma	
Sarcoma botryoides	
Neuroblastoma	
Blood clot	
Chronic granulomatous disease	
Radiation cystitis	

Boag GS, Nolan RL: Sonographic features of urinary bladder involvement in regional enteritis. J Ultrasound Med 7:125, 1988.

Friedman AP, Haller JO, Schulze G, et al.: Sonography of vesical and perivesical abnormalities in children. J Ultrasound Med 2:385, 1983.

Miller WB, Boal DK, Teele R: Neurofibromatosis of the bladder: Sonographic findings. J Clin Ultrasound 11:460, 1983.

Shapeero LG, Vordermark JS: Bladder neurofibromatosis in childhood: Noninvasive imaging. J Ultrasound Med 9:177, 1990.

Suzuki T, Yasumoto M, Shibuya M, et al.: Sonography of cyclophosphamide hemorrhagic cystitis: A report of two cases. J Clin Ultrasound 16:183, 1988.

MASSES

Common

Blood clot
Foley balloon catheter
Debris from infection

Uncommon

Neurofibroma
Rhabdomyosarcoma
Sarcoma botryoides
Neuroblastoma
Prostatic rhabdomyosarcoma
Calculus
Ureterocele
Pheochromocytoma
Chloroma
Metastases
Foreign body
Fungus balls

Friedman AP, Haller JO, Schulze G, et al.: Sonography of vesical and perivesical abnormalities in children. J Ultrasound Med 2:385, 1983.
Shapeero LG, Vordermark JS: Bladder neurofibromatosis in childhood: Noninvasive imaging. J Ultrasound Med 9:177, 1990.

Pelvic Masses

PRESACRAL

	Comment
Sacrococcygeal teratoma	
Anterior meningocele	
Neurenteric cysts	
Chordoma	
Retrorectal cysts	
Ectopic kidney	
Neuroblastoma	
Ganglioneuroma	
Neurofibroma	
Abscess	
Ulcerative colitis	Uterus/vagina
Osteomyelitis (sacrum)	
Sacral bone tumors	
Retroperitoneal sarcomas	

Miller WB, Boal DK, Teele R: Neurofibromatosis of the bladder: Sonographic findings. J Clin Ultrasound 11:460, 1983.

Haller HO: Pediatric pelvic ultrasound, in Sarti D: *Diagnostic Ultrasound: Text and Cases*, 2nd ed. Chicago, Year Book Medical Publishers, Inc., 1987, p 1146.

RECTOVESICAL

Common	Comment
Appendiceal abscess	
PID	
Normal female organ	Ovaries, uterus, or vagina
Lymphadenopathy	

Uncommon

Ureterocele	
Massive hydroureter	
Teratoma	
Diverticulum (bladder)	
Hydrosalpinx	
Ovarian cyst	
Lymphosarcoma	
Rhabdomyosarcoma	Sarcoma botryoides
Yolk sac carcinoma	
Hydrometrocolpos / hydrocolpos	
Foreign body abscess (vaginal perforation)	
Leukemic masses	
Neurofibroma	
Lymphangioma	Complex with anechoic portions
Müllerian duct cyst	In males
Fluid in cul-de-sac	Ascites or CSF from shunt
Blood in cul-de-sac	

Miller WB, Boal DK, Teele R: Neurofibromatosis of the bladder: Sonographic findings. J Clin Ultrasound 11:460, 1983.

Pretorius DH, Drose JA, Dennis MA, et al.: Tracheoesophageal fistula in utero: Twenty-two cases. J Ultrasound Med 6:509, 1987.

Shirkhoda A, Eftekhari F, Frankel LS, et al.: Diagnosis of leukemic relapse in the pelvic soft tissues of juvenile females. J Clin Ultrasound 14:191, 1986.

MALE

	Comment
Fluid	Ascites, blood, or CSF from shunt
Teratoma	
Seminal vesicle cyst	
Utricle cyst	Region of prostate
Bladder diverticulum	
Rhabdomyosarcoma of prostate	
Prostate abscess	
Duplication cyst of bowel	
Undescended testicle	
Pars infravaginalis gubernaculum	Bulbous termination of cord from testis to scrotum; may see mass in undescended testis
Müllerian duct cyst	Extends from prostate
Ectopic kidney	
Abscess, any cause	

Gregg DC, Sty JR: Sonographic diagnosis of enlarged prostatic utricle. J Ultrasound Med 8:51, 1989.
Rosenfield AR, Blair DN, McCarthy S, et al.: The pars infravaginalis gubernaculi: Importance in the identification of the undescended testis. AJR 153:775, 1989.

Ovaries and Adnexa

CYSTS

Common

Primordial follicles
Follicular cysts
Torsion of ovary
Endometrioma
Ectopic pregnancy

Comment

Common in early adolescence

Enlarged ovary

Uncommon

Teratoma
Teratocarcinoma
Dysgerminoma
Leukemic infiltration
Metastases
Cystadenoma
Cystadenocarcinoma
Pancreatic pseudocyst
Postoperative seroma
Enteric duplication cyst
Polycystic ovaries
Hydrosalpinx
PID
Abscess, any cause

Unusual before age 20

Graif M, Itzchak Y: Sonographic evaluation of ovarian torsion in childhood and adolescence. AJR 150:647, 1988.

Gupta AK, Berry M, Bhargava S: Sonographic double target in a case of type Ia cecal duplication cyst. J Clin Ultrasound 15:273, 1987.

Helvie MA, Silver TM: Ovarian torsion: Sonographic evaluation. J Clin Ultrasound 17:327, 1989.

Sherer DM, Shah YG, Eggers PC, et al.: Prenatal sonographic diagnosis and subsequent management of fetal adnexal torsion. J Ultrasound Med 9:161, 1990.

MASSES, SOLID OR COMPLEX

Common

	Comment
Torsion of ovary	Enlarged ovary; usually with cysts
Ectopic pregnancy	
Appendiceal abscess	
Tubo-ovarian abscess	
Lymphadenopathy	

Uncommon

Teratoma	Hypoechoic or hyperechoic or mixed
Teratocarcinoma	
Dysgerminoma	May be cystic or complex
Leukemic infiltration	
Metastases	
Cystadenoma	Usually cystic
Rhabdomyosarcoma	
Lymphoma	Usually hypoechoic
Endometrioma	Frequently has complex appearance
Cystadenocarcinoma	
Leukemic masses	
Lymphangioma	Complex appearance with anechoic portions

Pancreatic pseudocyst
Duplicated uterus with unilateral
  hematometrocolpos
Ectopic kidney
Abscess, any cause

Blumhagen JD, Wood BJ, Rosenbaum DM: Sonographic evaluation of abdominal lymphangiomas in children. J Ultrasound Med 6:487, 1987.

Graif M, Itzchak Y: Sonographic evaluation of ovarian torsion in childhood and adolescence. AJR 150:647, 1988.

Helvie MA, Silver TM: Ovarian torsion: Sonographic evaluation. J Clin Ultrasound 17:327, 1989.

Ngo C, Verma RC, Wong L, et al.: Simulation of a hydronephrotic pelvic kidney by an unusual pelvic mass. J Clin Ultrasound 15:126, 1987.

Sherer DM, Shah YG, Eggers PC, et al.: Prenatal sonographic diagnosis and subsequent management of fetal adnexal torsion. J Ultrasound Med 9:161, 1990.

Sheth S, Fishman EK, Buck JL, et al.: The variable sonographic appearances of ovarian teratomas: Correlation with CT. AJR 151:331, 1988.

Shirkhoda A, Eftekhari F, Frankel LS, et al.: Diagnosis of leukemic relapse in the pelvic soft tissues of juvenile females. J Clin Ultrasound 14:191, 1986.

Testes, Scrotum, and Epididymis

ENLARGED TESTES

	Comment
Orchitis	Focal or generalized hypoechogenicity
Acute torsion (after 24h)	Hypoechoic
Subacute torsion (1-10 degrees)	Hypoechoic
Idiopathic macroorchidism	
Masses	Can't differentiate; usually focally hypoechoic
Embryonal cell carcinoma	
Seminomas	
Teratomas	
Rhabdomyosarcoma	
Leydig's cell tumor	
Sertoli's cell tumor	
Metastases	Neuroblastoma
Leukemia/lymphoma	Inhomogeneous echogenicity
Trauma	

Albert NE: Testicular ultrasound for trauma. J Urol 124:558, 1980.
Bird K, Rosenfield AT, Taylor KJW: Ultrasonography in testicular torsion. Radiology 147:527, 1983.
Sample WF, Gottesman JE, Skinner DG, et al.: Gray scale ultrasound of the scrotum. Radiology 127:225, 1978.
Truwit CL, Jackson M, Thompson IM: Idiopathic macroorchidism. J Clin Ultrasound 17:200, 1989.

SMALL TESTES

	Comment
Chronic torsion	Hypoechoic
Undescended testicle	Hypoechoic
Postinfection atrophy	

Bird K, Rosenfield AT, Taylor KJW: Ultrasonography in testicular torsion. Radiology 147:527, 1983.
Wolverson MK, Houttuin E, Heiberg E, et al.: Comparison of computed tomography with high-resolution real time ultrasound in the localization of the impalpable undescended testis. Radiology 146:133, 1983.

ENLARGED SCROTUM

Hydrocele
Hematocele
Epididymo-orchitis
Torsion
Testicular tumor
Extratesticular tumor

MASS, EXTRATESTICULAR

Adenomatoid tumor of epididymis
Epididymal cyst
Utricle cyst
Hematoma
Adrenal rests
Spermatocele
Varicocele
Cyst of tunica albuginea

ENLARGED EPIDIDYMIS

Epididymitis
Adenomatoid tumor
Torsion

Acronyms and Abbreviations

ADKD   adult polycystic kidney disease

AIDS   acquired immune deficiency syndrome

APVR   anomalous pulmonary venous return

A-V canal   atrioventricular canal

AVM   arteriovenous malformation

BPH   benign prostatic hypertrophy

CCAM   congenital cystic adenomatoid malformation

CHARGE (association)   coloboma (eye), heart disease, choanal atresia, retarded growth and development (with or without CNS anomalies), genital hypoplasia, ear anomalies (with or without deafness); 2 or more needed to make the diagnosis

CHF   congestive heart failure

CML   chronic myelocytic leukemia

CMV (infection)   cytomegalovirus

CNS   central nervous system

CSF   cerebrospinal fluid

ECMO   extracorporeal membranous oxygen

ESWL   extracorporeal shock wave lithotripsy

IgA   immunoglobulin A

GI   gastrointestinal

GU   genitourinary

IPKD   infantile polycystic kidney disease

IUD   intrauterine device

IUGR   intrauterine growth retardation

IUP   intrauterine pregnancy

IVC   inferior vena cava

PID   pelvic inflammatory disease

PS   pulmonary stenosis

RLQ   right lower quadrant

RV   right ventricle

SBE   subacute bacterial endocarditis

TAPVR   total anomalous pulmonary venous return

TB   tuberculosis

T-E fistula   tracheoesophageal fistula

TGC (curves)   time gain compensation

TORCH   toxoplasmosis, other (viruses), rubella, CMV, herpes (simplex viruses)

TPN   total parenteral nutrition

UPJ   ureteropelvic junction

UVJ   ureterovesical junction

VSD   ventricular septal defect